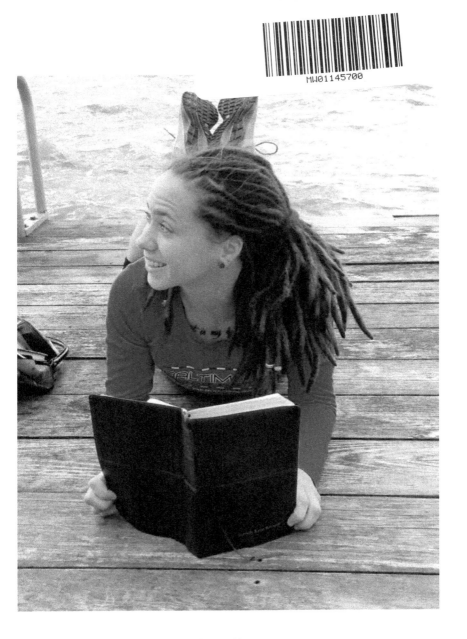

www.GabrielleRenee.org

GABRIELLE REHMEYER

RANSOMED HEART

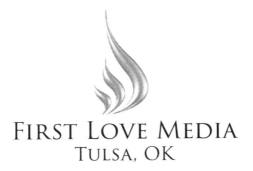

FIRST LOVE MEDIA
Tulsa, OK

Ransomed Heart
Coming Out of Homosexuality and Into the Father's Arms
Published by First Love Media
Tulsa, OK
www.FirstLoveMedia.com

ISBN 978-0-98305-352-1

Printed in the United States of America

DEDICATION

This book is dedicated firstly to my Savior. You have asked me to write and I have no choice but to obey for the love You have shown and continue to show me, how can I do anything else. My sincere hope and prayer is that in doing so, those who find themselves in a similar struggle, families of those who are struggling, and those who do not even realize yet that they are struggling, might be encouraged, might encounter You as You pursue each and every one of their hearts. Just as You pursued mine even as I wandered in the dark completely oblivious, for many years, to the extent of my brokenness.

I would also like to dedicate this book to my family. I know I put you through more pain than I like to recount. I know I hurt you. I know at times you did not know how to respond to the person I became. But I thank you for standing in the gap for me. I thank you for being strong enough to love me, though my actions and words were enough to turn anyone away. I thank you for your consistent prayer and for being close, while far away, over this past year as I have and am still learning who I am in Him. I love you guys with all of my heart and I am so thankful that when God initially authored this story, He decided to make me your daughter and big sister.

Table of Contents

Acknowledgements..09

Foreword..13

Prologue..17

1. The American Dream..25

2. Umboso weSwatini..31

3. Ladies Don't Play Football...41

4. A Whole New World...47

5. Running Out of Hiding...57

6. Home of the Free...65

7. Too Much and Never Enough..69

8. If You Are Not Real..73

9. He Simply Said Guard Your Heart...81

10. Now That I've Got Your Attention.......................................87

11. #WhiteGirlDreads..95

12. It Has All Become Too Much...103

13. What Was Meant for Evil..109

14. The Return..115

15. Fight..123

16. A New Name...135

17. Life Now...141

Epilogue..155

ACKNOWLEDGEMENTS

I have told my story, in bits and pieces, to numerous people. But these past eight years are difficult for me to write about- talking is easier for some reason. Writing has always been my 'thing'. I can write you a poem or a paragraph on how I am feeling- feelings- those I can write. I can put words together, I've been told, and I am thankful for this gift God has given me.

But this story. Has had my heart in knots, it makes me feel vulnerable, and quite honestly takes me to places and people that I do not want to revisit- the pain and the love is still very fresh. It pierces a place in my heart that for so many years was the only identity I allowed myself to know, or rather to painfully create. Yet, He will not let me get away from it. I can't even count the number of times someone has asked me to write, or the number of times I've heard the song "Write Your Story" by Francesca Battistelli, during moments where God brings it to my mind and heart. (Okay, okay, God…I'll listen). Please bear with me as I try to get this down on paper.

First, I would like to give thanks.

I cannot begin to thank Him enough for the grace He has shown me. For His pursuit of my heart, no matter how many times I denied and rebuked and intentionally spat in His face.

Jesus, I will never, ever comprehend Your love for me. And I've given up trying to. I simply rest in knowing You never let me go. And Your plans are higher and bigger and wider and deeper than I ever imagined. Please speak, write, move through me. Use me, Father.

I could write pages about how thankful I am. I sometimes am in disbelief that I am in this place now. There have been many key people who have not ceased in speaking truth into my life, though when I was in the middle of it all I was too blind and angry to see it that way. My sincerest apologies for my, at times not so kind, words and actions. I have learned that love speaks truth, always. And many times truth does offend, especially when we are in the wrong. We don't like to be corrected. I am so thankful for the gentle correction of the Holy Spirit in my life even when I thought I had completely blocked Him out.

For those of you, family and friends, who reached out to me over the past years as God led you to do so, I may not have been in a place to thank you then, but seeds were planted. Thank you for your obedience. To my prayer warriors around the world, those I know and those I do not yet have the honor of knowing, I thank you. Prayer is powerful. You taught me that. I thank you all for interceding on my behalf. To my sisi, Jacci- you've been a big sister to me since before all of this began. You went through all of this with my family just as if you were truly one of us, and you could never understand how much that means to me. I look up to you and am thankful that through all of this, you, were there and loved me even when I pushed you away. To my prayer warrior and spiritual mom, Doreen, your wisdom and leadership have meant more to me than you know. Thank you for pushing me to begin writing this book. Sister Ose, thank you for ministering into my life and for continuing to encourage me to grow in our Savior, for teaching me the importance of healing, no matter how much the process hurts.

To my best friend and twin, Heather, I am so honored to have been able to go through all of this with you. He is getting an army ready, and I am so thankful I get to fight this with you as your sister in Christ. To all who have mentored me this past year: Adeola, Iyanu, and Gabi, I love you guys. Your selflessness and willingness to stop what you are doing to pray for and with us, to talk sense into us, to correct us, and to love and guide us no matter what time of the day or night, has shown me, truly, what it means to be a servant leader as Jesus demonstrated. You have become family. And to my church family at CAC Bethel and BCF: Thank you for showing love and strength in vulnerability, in not being afraid to share where you came from, what you struggle with, and most importantly, what Christ has done in your lives. Your hunger for Christ is evident, and I am honored to belong to this family of world-changers.

Lord give me wisdom and conviction in everything I say and do, every choice I make, every interaction every moment I spend in the company of any and every one... May it have purpose. May my words never be uttered to simply fill silence. Speak through me. Teach me to know Your voice more clearly than I know my own. And teach me to obey. Even when I don't understand. Break my heart for what breaks Yours. Lead me. Guide me. Be forever in front and beside me. I long to live a life of purpose, in constant and unbroken fellowship with You, living the life You intended before I even existed

Foreword by Ose Burnett

There are times and events in our lives that are life-changing. They come through different stages; happy events, tragic events, traumatic events. So many defining moments that can paint a tapestry of our identity and destiny. And many times, people view our lives from a perspective that is surface-based. They see you every day, and they know how you like your coffee in the morning when you come to work. They laugh with you at church, and see the tears fall as you worship God with such fervency and love. They see how your family interacts with each other, and they envy the love that you have for one another. But they don't really know the whole story. They only know in part. They only know the story they have created in their mind about you. But they really don't know you.

When I met Gabrielle, I didn't know the whole story. All I knew was that she was loved furiously by Jesus, and He wanted to make sure that she knew that. So He had me come to her church to pray for her and her friend. I didn't know her story, but Jesus did. What transpired in that room was glorious. He alone knew her story. He knew her heartbreak. He knew her battle with homosexuality. He knew all of it. And He just loved her. He loved her so much, that He wrapped His arms around her, and told her that over and over, and over again. It was an amazing encounter with the amazing God of the universe, and His Son, Jesus.

Months later, she texts me and asks me to read her book, and I did. What I didn't realize was that I was reading her story. Her story of redemption. I read it with awe and excitement, and trepidation. When I was done, the first thought that came to mind was, "She will be persecuted for this book." The second thought was, "Millions will be delivered from the homosexual lifestyle because of this book." The second thought outweighed the first, and it was then I was excited, and showed it to my husband. And now we are here.

Gabrielle's life is not what many would expect from a missionary's daughter. Many would think that being raised in a Christian home would exempt you from the attacks of the devil. It is far from truth. And that's why her story is even more remarkable. It could have ended much, much worse. But the fact that the Word of God was sown into her life, is a testament to parents and grandparents everywhere, that you should never give up on praying for your loved ones. *God still answers prayers*, and for those of you who have loved ones in this lifestyle, this book is a tool of evangelism. Give it to them as the Lord leads. Gabrielle understands exactly what drew her to the arms of a woman, and how her identity was stolen from her by the enemy. You will see through her eyes the hunger that many have to be free from this lifestyle. Do not believe that they are happy to be in this lifestyle. It is a deception that is being pushed by the media, by schools, and the government. We have the answer.

Gabrielle is not alone. There are countless more that have the exact same story. The Lord has given her the boldness to write this book, so that many will come to know the saving power of the gospel of Jesus Christ. As you read this book,

I pray that you will come to know the love of Jesus, and His desire to be in every aspect of your life. He loves you, just as much as He loves Gabrielle. Get to know His love today.

PROLOGUE

My mom was here for my college graduation in May of this year. She brought back a stack of journals, seven to be exact, dating back to March 6th, 2004. The very first journal entry I ever wrote was after middle school youth group, Pathfinders, when Pastor Chad Daniel preached and prophesied that I was called to be a full time minister. Who, me?! Needless to say- I was a little bit passionate. He clearly must have heard wrong, though, because I had already made other plans, and while being in missions was on this blueprint, it surely was not a full-time position.

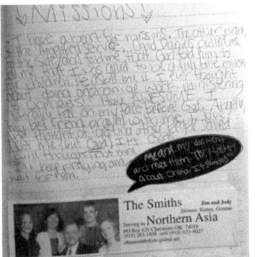

It has been the craziest thing to be able to look back through seven journals- documenting my life as a very passionate and soccer obsessed 13 year old up until I stopped writing in 2008. Looking at my early journals makes me laugh because I was, and maybe still am just a little tiny bit, a drama queen. So for your entertainment and so you can see where my priorities were during my early years, I have included some pictures of journal entries, including #6 on my 13-year-old self's 'Stress List':

"I used to think I had everything planned…Maybe God does have a bigger plan for my life than I do. Maybe His plan is completely different from mine. Maybe I am supposed to be a missionary. I don't know. CONFUSED."

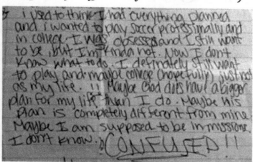

Though funny, this and many other entries have opened my eyes to a number of things. Firstly: I knew at a young age that His calling on my life was bigger than I could fathom. Secondly: I was slightly obsessed with soccer. Thirdly: I was passionately in love with Jesus Christ. But I was unsure of myself, and I had no idea how to combine and balance the above priorities. I remember watching movies as a child and thinking, "wow, I wish that could happen in real life" or "why can't my life be this interesting?" I feel like God was listening (not that He's never not listening) and I imagine Him responding with, "If only you could see what is to come, if only you could see what I see."

This book explains my journey so far, granted, I only have 25 years under my belt. It started off pretty boring, or so I thought. As mentioned, my life consisted of soccer and Jesus, in that order. The next thing I knew we were in Africa, and the struggle for my identity took a turn I never imagined. This struggle was more than I could bear and I eventually stopped fighting. I hurt my family, denied and rebuked the God I once loved, and eventually made it my goal and purpose to fight for a lifestyle that had become the focal point of my identity. And through it all, Jesus never stopped fighting on my behalf.

This story is more than my story; it is another example of the saving grace of Jesus. It is a story of how He pursued a very lost and broken heart, yet one He ransomed on the cross so many years ago. It is a story that keeps telling, as He continues to teach me what walking and living with Him looks like since He has called me out of homosexuality and into His embrace. It is a story of a war that waged in a realm I could not see, but so deeply felt.

Most importantly, it is a story of victory, a message of hope for anyone who may be fighting a similar battle. As with any sin, this battle is not one that ends the day you surrender your life to Christ, or at least mine didn't play out this way. And in the midst of my struggle I prayed and hoped for someone to come into my life who had been through something similar. I heard plenty of stories of those who came "out of the closet", and was congratulated for being brave enough to come out of my own, but deep down I longed to meet someone who had come out of this lifestyle.

One thing I have learned, the hard way, is that it is impossible to walk away in your own strength. This is not a physical battle. It is not a mind game where if you concentrate hard enough on not thinking about or not doing certain things, you will be free from it. Trying is in vain if He is not involved. And while I believe wholeheartedly in the word of God, this is not a book drilling what the Bible says regarding homosexuality. If you want a sound theological study of this, there are a good number of books out there explaining homosexuality from a Biblical perspective (I would recommend What Does the Bible Really Teach about Homosexuality? by Kevin DeYoung and Can You Be Gay and Christian by Dr. Michael Brown).

Since the fall of man, we have all been born into sin and iniquity. Some of us may be prone to certain sinful behaviors and patterns. For many, certain sins were introduced to us and due to having certain areas of our lives not surrendered to the Holy Spirit, the Enemy took advantage and we found ourselves struggling with something that may have shocked us. Whatever the case may be, because of Christ dying on the cross and raising from the dead, reconciling us to the Father, we do not have to dwell in sin. Though it may not be easy, there is always a choice involved. The Bible rebukes all sin. No one sin is worse or greater than another. Homosexuality is one of many, and it happened to be my struggle. The kid you sit next to in church who tells a lie to his mom is just as guilty as the person who engages in homosexual activity. Both can be repented of, and both can turn into a lifestyle if not surrendered to Jesus.

The reason there is a difference, I believe, is that homosexuality deals with your identity. And it is increasingly not only condoned, but celebrated and encouraged. One would not approach you and identify themselves as a liar, or a fornicator, or a murderer. However, the acts of lying, fornicating, murdering, and homosexual intimacy are all sin, and the person is still guilty before God, regardless of whether or not these sins are celebrated by man. Embracing homosexuality involves turning away from God's order and design (Genesis 2:24). In a sense, it is an attempt, rooted in pride, to be god, to re-make the rules, our actions telling God that His creation and design is not good. So I will mention the key verses here and not repeat them in the remainder of the book.

    1. *Do not practice homosexuality, having sex with another man as with a woman. It is a detestable sin (Leviticus 18:22, NLT).*

    2. *If a man practices homosexuality, having sex with another man as with a woman, both men have committed a detestable act. They must both be put to death, for they are guilty of a capital offense (Leviticus 20:13, NLT).*

    Though Old Testament, the Holiness Code is still relevant and should be taken seriously as they reflect the holy character of God and give us insight to what is expected for us to be holy. The law is Holy and righteous and good (Romans 7). We were not able to keep the law by our own might or strength, but we also could not fellowship with a Holy God while we were living in sin, which explains the severity of the punishment. He is as much a God of Justice as He is of Love. Thank God for Jesus bridging that gap and becoming the ultimate sacrifice so that in spite of ourselves, we can still have access to the Father.

    3. *For since the creation of the world His invisible attributes are clearly seen, being understood by the things that are made, even His eternal power and Godhead, so that they are without excuse, because, although they knew God, they did not glorify Him as God, nor were thankful, but became futile in their thoughts, and their foolish hearts were darkened. Professing to be wise, they became fools, and changed the glory of the incorruptible God into an image made like corruptible man--and birds and four-footed animals and creeping things. Therefore God also gave them up to uncleanness, in the lusts of their hearts, to dishonor their bodies among themselves, who exchanged the truth of God for the lie, and worshiped and served the creature rather than the Creator, who is blessed forever.*

Amen. For this reason God gave them up to vile passions. For even their women exchanged the natural use for what is against nature. Likewise also the men, leaving the natural use of the woman, burned in their lust for one another, men with men committing what is shameful, and receiving in themselves the penalty of their error which was due. And even as they did not like to retain God in their knowledge, God gave them over to a debased mind, to do those things which are not fitting; being filled with all unrighteousness, sexual immorality, wickedness, covetousness, maliciousness; full of envy, murder, strife, deceit, evil-mindedness; they are whisperers, backbiters, haters of God, violent, proud, boasters, inventors of evil things, disobedient to parents, undiscerning, untrustworthy, unloving, unforgiving, unmerciful; who, knowing the righteous judgment of God, that those who practice such things are deserving of death, not only do the same but also approve of those who practice them (Romans 1:20-32, NIV).

4. *Don't you realize that those who do wrong will not inherit the Kingdom of God? Don't fool yourselves. Those who indulge in sexual sin, or who worship idols, or commit adultery, or are male prostitutes, or practice homosexuality, or are thieves, or greedy people, or drunkards, or are abusive, or cheat people— none of these will inherit the Kingdom of God. Some of you were once like that. But you were cleansed; you were made holy; you were made right with God by calling on the name of the Lord Jesus Christ and by the Spirit of our God. You say, "I am allowed to do anything"—but not everything is good for you. And even though "I am allowed to do anything," I must not become a slave to anything. You say, "Food was made for the stomach, and the stomach for food." (This is true, though someday God will do away with both of them.) But you can't say that our bodies were made for sexual immorality. They were made for the Lord, and*

the Lord cares about our bodies. And God will raise us from the dead by his power, just as he raised our Lord from the dead (1 Corinthians 6:9-14, NLT),

5. *We know that the law is good when used correctly. For the law was not intended for people who do what is right. It is for people who are lawless and rebellious, who are ungodly and sinful, who consider nothing sacred and defile what is holy, who kill their father or mother or commit other murders. The law is for people who are sexually immoral, or who practice homo-sexuality, or are slave traders, liars, promise breakers, or who do anything else that contradicts the wholesome teaching that comes from the glorious Good News entrusted to me by our blessed God (1 Timothy 1:8-11, NLT).*

I don't believe one simply comes out or walks away from this lifestyle. If I had not been called out, drawn out, carried out, at first kicking and screaming, if I had not encountered Jesus, there is no way I would be where I am today. I did not simply walk away and never look back. I was pursued. And I am so thankful He loved me enough to not give up on me. I would have given up on me. He is a good, good Father, and there is reason for everything He has said we should and should not do, even when we do not see or understand. It took me learning to trust His heart, rather than my very flawed and fleeting emotions.

> *My child, don't reject the LORD's discipline,*
> *and don't be upset when he corrects you.*
> *For the LORD corrects those he loves,*
> *just as a father corrects a child in whom he delights*
> *(Proverbs 3:11-12, NLT).*

Today, I walk with Jesus, with a changed heart, perspective, and desires that I pray daily would align with His. But it has been a journey getting to this place of peace and joy, and is one that is continuing even as I write this very sentence, through daily surrender and submission to Him. My prayer is that this testimony can be the very one I yearned to hear, in your own life.

CHAPTER 1: THE AMERICAN DREAM

My mom grew up in the Pentecostal church- Assemblies of God, to be exact, and if you were to ask my dad, she was born saved. He, on the other hand, not so much. My parents met at Family Worship Center, in Baton Rouge, Louisiana, in 1988, the day that Brother Jimmy Swaggart confessed to his congregation and those listening worldwide that he had sinned, asking forgiveness. On this day, my dad's boss convinced him to go to church with her. My mom was sitting in the balcony on this 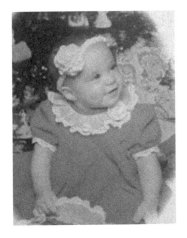 particular night, and watched as my dad surrendered his life to Christ at the altar, though she did not yet know him. This was February of 1988. They were married at Family Worship Center in December of that same year. I was the first born, in 1991, followed by two sisters and one brother.

My mom, a nurse, and my dad, an engineer, we were your

typical middle class American family. At least, I think we were. As far as I know, we were, but then all I have to judge by is what I saw on TV and the other families we were surrounded by. From the time my dad became a Christian, he felt the call to the mission field, but could not seem to figure out how to align reality with the longing in his heart. He had my siblings and I involved in outreach from a young age as my parents led a street ministry- 'Street Jam', where on Saturday mornings, we would take a trailer that opened up into a stage to the inner city of Baton Rouge. Here, we would have worship, puppet shows, and my dad would preach. For a period of time my dad felt that we would be missionaries to South America.

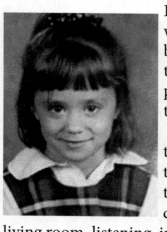

I remember attending Spanish lessons with him many evenings after school, because I wanted to be a missionary too (and I enjoyed showing off my pronunciation, which was much better than his).

Missionary families from all over the world would return to the States to visit and my dad must have been on the contact list, because I would frequently find myself sitting in someone's living room, listening, in wide-eyed complete amazement as they would speak on what it was like to live in China and preach the Gospel. I was fascinated. I wanted this. But it felt more like a dream. It was someone else's life; I couldn't really imagine my family packing everything up, leaving everyone behind and answering this call. I had an imagination, and I definitely believed that I would one day be a missionary- after school and college and my professional soccer career, and maybe after I had spent a few years as a secret agent in the

CIA. Again, it seemed just as real to me as these other dreams.

Though I was constantly in church, I had a rebellious spirit and control issues from a very early age. I could be a handful, to put it lightly. Throughout preschool and elementary school I was constantly in trouble for bullying other kids, whether it be forcing someone to eat dirt, or forcing someone to embrace a stinging caterpillar (not sure how I pulled that one off). Noises bothered me, and when I was little I couldn't understand that when someone made a noise such as sniffling or coughing, they usually could not help it and were not doing so to purposefully get on my nerves. Therefore, anyone who got on my nerves, was either pinched, bitten, or threatened.

Needless to say, my mom was often times not sure what to do with me and would have to leave work to pick me up from school, in tears because I had threatened yet another child that if they returned to school the next day I would kill them. Yes, kill. Did I mean it? Most definitely not. Did I have issues? Clearly.

To my parents, and my classmates' parents' great relief, I grew out of this, or at least learned to control it: distraction, copy the behavior (kind of like a reset button), or simply walk away and recuperate. We all have our peculiarities.

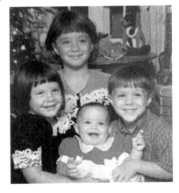

Up until around middle school, we remained at Family Worship Center. I loved going to church as a child, which was good I suppose, since we were there Wednesdays, Sunday mornings and evenings, and sometimes multiple days in a row if it was Camp Meeting. I looked forward to Camp Meeting and to Kids' Camp, because I got to meet kids from all over the country, and mostly because I loved to worship. At around 7 years old I gave my heart to Jesus at an altar call at a Camp Meeting children's service- "Salvation Station". I was filled with the Holy Spirit around this age too and remember very clearly the first time I spoke in tongues.

Right before I started the 6th grade we started attending a church called Healing Place, also in Baton Rouge. Here, I was able to become more involved in youth group, and there were more mission opportunities, which was one of the reasons we moved. However, soccer had very quickly become priority in the Rehmeyer household once I began playing premier soccer, which was basically more competitive than playing recreational (more expensive, more time intensive, and more pressure). My sister and brother also joined the premier league and once there were 3 of us playing, our every evening and weekend was spent at the soccer fields, either in Baton Rouge or at tournaments in neighboring states.

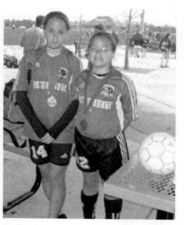

With our lives consumed with soccer and my parents working nonstop to try to afford this, things became quite tense during my pre-teen years. I have countless journal entries from this time with petitions to God regarding "the Discover card bill", which must have been a hot topic in our house. My dad finally had enough and knew there must be more to life than what ours had become. One Sunday morning, there was a missionary couple at church representing an organization called Children's Cup, based in Swaziland, Africa. After the service, my dad spoke with them to inquire about how my family might be able to be involved with missions, even if that meant stuffing envelopes or doing whatever odd job that was needed in order to be some sort of help.

Slightly different from stuffing envelopes, a few weeks later, my parents left us in the care of my grandparents and were on their way to Swaziland. During the time they were away, I was reading a book called 'The Dream Giver' by Bruce Wilkinson. God really spoke to my heart through this book. He was preparing me for Swaziland at the same time He was working wonders in my mom's heart. She was dead-set against leaving our comfortable life in Baton Rouge, and assured everyone that she was only going to make my dad happy so that he would stop talking about it.

While they were away, I sat my three younger siblings down and told them, "We're going to move to Swaziland, so don't be scared when mom and dad tell us; it's going to be okay." They were 10, 9, and 6 at the time. Surely enough, my parents returned from Swaziland, sure of where God was calling them. Unknown to me at the time, they were only waiting for Him to confirm this incredible move through their 4 children, who they did not think would be up to being uprooted and moved to the other side of the world. My mom said she spent the entirety of the trip completely overwhelmed with emotion because of the clarity with which God was speaking to her heart regarding moving to Swaziland.

When they sat us down to tell us the news, before they could even get a word in, I spoke up, "Mom, Dad, I think we need to move to Swaziland." And with that, my parents set a goal to be in Swaziland within 9 months. Acting in faith, they did not enroll us into school the next year, trusting that God was going to provide the money and everything else we needed to follow through with His plan. The next 9 months were incredibly busy: my mom left her job; my dad sold his business; we sold our cars, and had the biggest garage sale in the history of garage sales (or any I have seen).

In August of 2005 we still did not have the funding we needed to make the move, but acting in faith yet again, my parents went ahead and bought 6 one way tickets to Swaziland. Shortly after this, the funding came through, and we left Louisiana to head towards Maryland, where we would be flying out of, one day before hurricane Katrina demolished our home state in September of 2005. Talk about a lot going on.

Were we excited? Quite. Scared? Terrified. My biggest concern, of course: *How am I going to be a professional soccer player now?*

But Jesus, I trust you.

CHAPTER 2: Umbuso weSwatini

Nkulunkulu Mnikati wetibusiso temaSwati;
Siyatibonga tonkhe tinhlanhla,
Sibonga iNgwenyama yetfu,
Live netintsaba nemifula.

Busisa tiphatsimandla takaNgwane
Nguwe wedvwa Somandla wetfu;
Sinike kuhlakanipha lokungenabucili
Simise usicinise, Simakadze.

O Lord our God, bestower of the blessings of the Swazi;
We give Thee thanks for all our good fortune;
We offer thanks and praise for our King
And for our fair land, its hills and rivers.

Thy blessings be on all rulers of our Country;
Might and power are Thine alone;
We pray Thee to grant us wisdom without deceit or malice.
Establish and fortify us, Lord Eternal.

Above is the Swazi national anthem- which I learned
months after being in Swaziland, starting from humming

the tune, to being able to mumble some rendition of what I thought the words sounded like. Finally learning the spelling and meaning of the words I was trying to sing in siSwati class helped, greatly. SiSwati is a beautiful language and one regret I have is not putting in more effort while living there to fully learn the language. Unfortunately, I had other priorities.

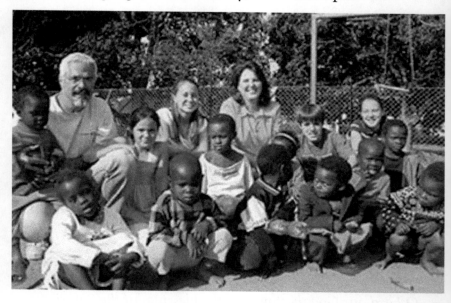

The move to Swaziland was tremendously exciting. We were moving from small town Baton Rouge, Louisiana where the most exciting thing was crawfish boils and our occasional monster hurricane, to Swaziland, Africa's only remaining absolute monarchy, ruled by King Mswati III, who (at the time) had around 12 wives. This beautifully mountainous country looked more like a movie scene compared to the completely flat and not so aesthetically pleasing environment we had grown up in.

However, at 13 years old, after a few weeks of being in this brand new country, after not having lived anywhere other than the one house in Baton Rouge, surrounded by very familiar family, friends, and routine, it hit me. We had just left all of the above and moved to the other side of the world. Not on a mission's trip. This was now home.

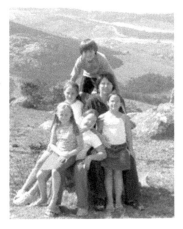

And it was incredibly expensive to make phone calls to the United States. Facebook wasn't what it has become, and skype may have been an option, if we had internet connection fast enough to allow such, which we did not. I cried myself to sleep for the first month or so, thinking about how much I missed my Mimi (my mom's mom) and Claire, who, was and still is my best friend, since the 6th grade.

Claire was the friend I cried to, the only person who understood my mood swings, and instead of returning the attitude, would warn people not to talk to me because "she is NOT a morning person". I was not always the nicest friend to Claire in middle school, those confusing years of trying to fit in and trying to be a cheerleader when you know you should just stick to soccer. But I would have done anything for Claire, and her, me. In fact, I distinctly remember kicking a certain boy in the face in Bible class in 6th grade, yes Bible class, because he said something about her I found to be offensive. I won't go into too much detail here, but he cried. I told him I would do it again if he didn't stop, and when the teacher asked what was wrong, he said he had a cold. Good answer. I told you I had issues.

Claire was not only my best friend and confidant, she

was my prayer warrior and my worship buddy. We did everything together. As I was going through a lot of change in Swaziland, so was she in the US. I looked forward to our daily email exchange. Her constant prayer and encouragement got me through some rough times, and I wish I would have been a better friend, even from the other side of the world, as she struggled, too.

I eventually made friends among other missionary families and church youth groups. I started running 10k and half marathons with some of the missionary guys in our community. It helped me worry less about the fact that I was most definitely losing all skill and hopes of becoming a professional soccer player with each passing day that I was not practicing my life away on the soccer field. I started school a few months after moving to Swaziland, at Waterford Kamhlaba UWC (United World College of Southern Africa), which was founded in 1963 in opposition to the apartheid system of education then being practiced in South Africa.

We were completely unaware that such an incredible school just happened to be located in Mbabane, Swaziland, 10 minutes away from where we would be living. The first time one of our missionary friends took my mom and I up the Waterford hill, to visit the community that would soon become home to me, I was completely dumbfounded. The Waterford campus is beautiful- and from the top of the hill you can look out over the mountains and see almost the entire city of Mbabane, unless it was a cloudy day, which limited one's sight to about a 10 feet radius, as we were engulfed in the clouds.

I started school in the last few weeks of the 3rd (final) term of form 2 right before final exams. Thankfully, I was given a pass for the exams since it would have been near impossible to memorize the entire map of Africa in geography, learn Swaziland history, and figure out what on earth anyone was doing in maths (yes, maths, not math). I learned very quickly that the American and British school systems are quite different, and having been top of my class with straight A's all throughout school prior to this, I had a hard time adjusting, particularly to maths and sciences, which were significantly more advanced than what I was used to.

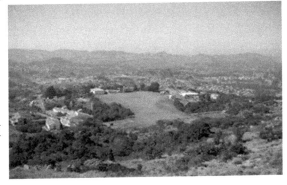

Thankfully, I made some wonderful friends who spent many hours working with me on topics I struggled with. Funny enough, I came out with an A in history, because while I struggled with the other classes and expected to not do so well, I was completely intrigued and spent many, many hours trying to soak in as much as I could about the history of this country that was now home. I figured I would just have to work hard to catch up with the other subjects once form 3 started.

While in Swaziland, I was still on fire for Christ. I led Bible studies at my school, wrote countless letters to friends and led many to the Lord. My ministry was in letter writing for a long time as I was scared to approach people, especially if I knew they swore a lot. I did not like the thought of being cussed out, so I would write pages and pages of how Jesus loves them and how He died for them. Lizzy, one of my good friends, who is now traveling the world as a missionary, came to the Lord through one of these letters and became a very special sister in Christ. One of my journal entries from this time reads: "God, if You would just give me a bus, I could bring all of my school friends to church and they would all get saved. I just need a bus because our car only seats 6 and 15 if we squeeze really tight."

I longed with all of my heart for my friends to experience Jesus the way I knew Him, but I also had never been to an International school surrounded by people from all around the world of all different beliefs and backgrounds. While many responded well to my zeal, others did not. It did not bother me at first. I was very passionate and headstrong and rather than tear me down, knowing someone was not a believer only made me more zealous to reach out.

I must admit, however, my tactics were at times not so mature, and I probably scared a few people away and offended others. For no other reason than I wanted to make a difference for Jesus. But I had no idea, none at all, of the storm that was coming my way. At this time in my life, through forms 2, 3, and 4, if you would have told me of the turn my life was going to take- I would have most definitely laughed in your face, and

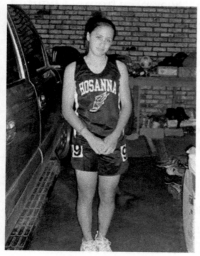

then asked if I could please pray for you.

Somewhere along the way I began to struggle with my identity, with my self-worth, with feelings of inadequacy. Granted, if I go back to even before we moved to Swaziland, this was something I had been struggling with for most of my adolescent years, the struggle was simply distracted by my soccer obsession and church activities. I very clearly remember being in middle school in Louisiana, running track, cross country and playing premier soccer, always doing some form of exercise, usually overdoing it, which landed me in physical therapy over and over again to the point where they stretched me so much I quite literally turned into Gumbi.

During the summer time when I was old enough to keep my siblings, I would force them to exercise as well- I termed it "boot camp". And they despised summers with me, of course. I was constantly self-conscious about the way I looked. In 6th and 7th grade I would ration myself to 4 crackers and 8 carrots a day, and I was always trying to control what everyone ate in my house, because it made me feel more in control of myself, I suppose. So, this identity struggle was not new for me, it simply looked different.

I had a few boyfriends and crushes in my pre-teen and early teenage years. The first was when I was in 8th grade, still in Louisiana. He was in 9th grade. It didn't last very long. I found him "giving guitar lessons" to a 12th grade girl in the chapel one day after school. Let's just say, it did not look like any guitar lesson I had ever seen. I was pretty heartbroken, but I got over it because the only person I ever truly loved (to the extent my heart was able, because yes, I loved him deeply), was my best friend's older brother. However, this was an interesting situation, which I will get to later.

Once in Swaziland, I had a few 'crushes' here and there, but the first guy I liked enough to say yes to girlfriend status, was and still is truly one of the most amazing guys I know. He has a heart of gold, and while he did not believe in the God I loved, he liked me so much that he would listen to me go on and on and on about Jesus and how much I loved Him. He would even suck it up and go to church with me, which I knew he didn't want to do. Though I began guitar lessons in the States about a year before moving to Swaziland, it was this particular guy who encouraged me to continue to play and taught me so much about music. I will be forever grateful for that. I eventually ended the relationship, though I liked him a lot, because I wanted to focus on my relationship with God and I knew my faith was not strong enough to be involved with someone who did not believe. He respected my decision, but for a long time, feelings remained on both sides.

Looking back, I didn't see the harm in casually dating or being in these relationships at this age. However, I realize now how each one truly did take a piece of my heart with it, despite how "unattached" I claimed to be. And if I were to go back, though I would be the same girl, with the same feelings and the same wandering heart, I would work on guarding it, because there are only so many pieces you can afford to lose before it begins to take a toll. However, this was only the beginning. A few years later I would be amazed at just how many pieces you can give away and still have anything left at all.

Lizzy and I took Waterford by storm. We had many mentors during our last years of high school, as many who were coming to Swaziland from the States were or were once youth pastors. They would come to share at our weekly Bible studies 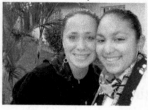 and help us get our friends excited about Jesus and coming down the hill to attend youth night on Fridays, or special events when ministry teams would come to speak. We felt covered as long as we had our youth pastors. However, no one stayed very long. When their time was up they had to go back home, and Lizzy and I struggled with feelings of abandonment and inadequacy and fear to be the light on our own.

There were others who stood up to lead with us, but when

I turned away I unfortunately led a few to turn with me. Lizzy stood tall and held on to Jesus with everything she had over the next few years. Our friendship would become strained, and would soon feel nonexistent as I made other friends and tried to avoid her at all costs. She would become a big sister to my siblings, who felt they had lost me. And she would write me letters, just as I had to her before she gave her life to Christ. I know she felt like she failed me during this time, but truthfully, I was not in a place to listen, and no matter how persistent anyone could have been, talking to me was like talking to a wall. The letters, however, got through to me when nothing and no one else could.

CHAPTER 3: LADIES DON'T PLAY FOOTBALL

Looking back in my journals, there was a distinct time where I felt God was asking me to give up something that had very much so be-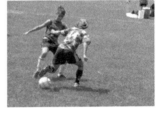come an idol. Soccer. There are places in my journals from Louisiana where I felt this was the case, but I couldn't do it. I practiced and practiced and went to all of the extra training sessions, to boys' team practices, to summer camps, and ODP (Olympic Developmental Program) tryouts every year, though I was never good enough to make the state team.

In Swaziland, I played soccer at school, but it was not as competitive as I was used to, so when my dad told me one day he had visited the Swaziland Women's Football Association and found a team I could join, I was beyond thrilled. I began playing for Imbabatane Ladies, sometimes referred to as Lady Swallows, as technically we were the sister team to the Mbabane Swallows (the capital city men's' team), though they never associated themselves or supported us, really. I take that back. There was that one time they donated their old uniforms that were about 3 sizes too big.

Playing for this league now meant I would be playing with and against the women who represented Swaziland on the national team, which I thought meant I was hot stuff, of course.

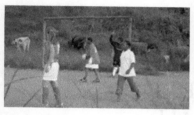

It also meant sometimes having games in the most interesting locations, such as prisons, or on dirt fields where the game would frequently be interrupted by a herd of friendly cows casually strolling through the field.

I quickly learned that culturally, in Swaziland, for women to play soccer was looked down upon, as a woman's place was at her homestead taking care of the family. Therefore, for many of the women on my team, who would soon become big sisters to me, playing soccer sometimes meant being disowned by their family. A few girls on my team actually lived with my coach, who understood the cost of playing, and was so passionate about our team that he would rather house them than lose them. I very quickly grew to love the ladies I played with, some of whom spoke only siSwati, and so the majority of what I learned in siSwati, I learned from time spent with them.

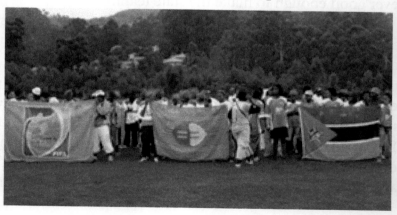

While I was used to being the best female soccer player up on the hill at Waterford, I quickly discovered that the skill level of many of the women I was now playing with and against greatly exceeded my own. They were like soccer goddesses to me. I had never seen women play soccer like this before. I lived for weekend games and tournaments in Mozambique and South Africa. Monday through Friday I would change into my soccer gear after classes, hop on the bus, and run from where the bus dropped us in town to where we practiced, which was a very small, uneven, half gravel, half dirt field behind some industrial buildings.

A few of the ladies on my team became like protective big 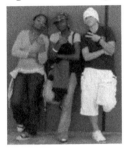 sisters to me, though I didn't quite understand why they felt the need to protect me at first. I absolutely loved it, though. I felt safe with them. And I was happy I was on their team because a few of my sisters, when provoked on the field, had been known to cause some damage. Eventually I did as well, as I learned to be more and more aggressive to compensate for the skill difference between myself and many of the women. My dad became our team transport and would somehow manage to fit an entire soccer team, plus the coach (at least 12 people) every weekend in a car that would legally and comfortably only seat 8. Hey, T.I.A (this is Africa). I suppose it was better than being crammed into the back of a pickup truck with the chickens and goats.

I lived to play soccer with these ladies. A little more urgent this time, I again felt God asking me to give up my idol. I refused. And soon after I was introduced to a whole new world that once seemed so foreign, but very quickly became my own. Though I was not fully aware of the changes going on inside my heart, of the numbness that was setting in as I began to harden my heart to His call and choose to pursue the path that was gratifying all the places in me that needed affirming, my outward appearance began to change. Most of the ladies I played with were very boy-like in appearance, in the way they carried themselves and dressed. I think for some, who were constantly told by everyone that soccer was for men and therefore they were trying be men, dressing the part seemed to be the way to go. I had always said I was a tom-boy, so I didn't think much of switching to boxers, baggy shorts, and beanies.

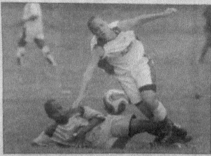

WOMEN'S FOOTBALL IS GOING PLACES

SOCCER – I wish to highlight the success that has been garnered by the recently concluded Shosholoza KFC Tournament.

It's so amazing how women's football is fast-gathering popularity and confidence among the sponsors. It's really a first that women's could succeed in bringing aboard a company like KFC to sponsor their games.

It really shows that women's football has come a long way to be what it is now and I have nothing but praise for those who have persisted.

Women's football is now a product worth selling to the people and I hope the Women's Football

getting to the top but it's more difficult staying there. This team has demonstrated a high degree of discipline and consistency by dominating women's football in the league with great aplomb.

What Correctional Services are doing in netball, Muchachas have shown that they can do it better in women's football. Now that they have started adding international accolades it shows that the team have got a long way to go.

And, make no mistake; the success is no means by miracle if you consider the toils by people like Esau du Pont. He has always been there behind the team and has shown that he has the talent to keep the team afloat.

Women's football is now a product worth selling.

CHAPTER 4: A WHOLE NEW WORLD

As I mentioned, the ladies I played with were mostly much older than me, and many gave me attention I had never experienced before. Not so much on my own team. Like I said, they were very protective over me and one in particular, who everyone called my sister due to her lighter complexion, was particularly protective. As the only white player in the women's league, I was receiving attention from both men and women soccer "stars" in the country, and even made my way into quite a few newspaper articles. This fed my insecurity, of course. It fed my feelings of inadequacy. It fed my pride. Then, the number one women's team in the country- the Muchachas, began trying to recruit me- I am

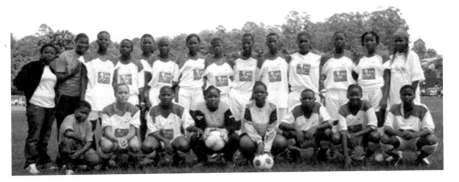

still not sure why, I had a pretty good left foot, but I was by no means comparable to some of the ladies on my team. But I felt honored and at one point thought about switching teams. I couldn't leave my team behind, so I would just quietly train with the Muchachas from time to time and guest play in tournaments.

While playing with Muchachas, I became very close friends with someone on the team. It started with me idolizing her because she was an incredible soccer player. I would make it a point to go to all of their games just to see her, and when I found out she was also in ministry at her church, I figured out how to get my family to welcome her into our home. Eventually when the other girls on our teams noticed we were spending so much time together they became jealous, and she became very territorial over me. She started to monitor who I would talk to and would become extremely angry if I gave anyone more attention than I was giving her. I started drinking and partying with some of the girls on her team, and began having to lie more and more to my parents in order to spend time with my new friends.

When I started to become scared of my own feelings towards her and other women, I contacted her pastor and his wife, and told them that I thought she was struggling with being a lesbian. Needless to say, that was pretty much the end of our friendship. I felt terrible and tried to apologize, unsuccessfully. Finally, just so she would speak to me again I admitted that it wasn't just her and that I was struggling too, but she never admitted to anything, so I was the one who got sent to counseling.

While all of this was happening, I had also become close friends with a girl at my church who was an up and coming rapper in Swaziland. She had admitted to me early on in our friendship that she liked girls and asked me if I would help her. I agreed to do so, though I was clearly already struggling myself, still completely oblivious of how deep I had already fallen. I had a boyfriend at this time, who I also met at church. We were all involved in youth leadership together, which soon became very difficult to juggle, because I eventually liked both of them and felt terrible because he was an incredible guy, and I was just as lost as lost could get.

There was one night that I remember very clearly, and also have written in one of my journals. We had a game night and sleepover at one of the American missionary's house, someone who was like a big sister to me. I had many 'big sisters and brothers' throughout my time in Swaziland. However, after a few years there I decided not to become close to anyone, because they never stayed as long as they said they would (and of course, I took it very personally).

This particular night, there was a lady who was on a short term mission's trip to Swaziland, who had shared (not with me) that she had struggled with homosexuality, but that God delivered her. She had a dream earlier during her time in Swaziland and seeing me that night confirmed what God was showing her. That night she told my big sister she sensed a very familiar spirit and that it was trying to make its way into my life. At the time, this would have sounded just as crazy as I'm sure it sounds to some of you reading this, which is probably why no one told me until later. I would have laughed, though my spirit would have most definitely resonated.

In fact, I remember looking at her and wondering what her story was. When I saw her, I saw hope, but I wasn't sure why. It was around this time I was dangerously close to the edge of the cliff, but I had not yet completely made the jump. I still hated the feelings that would rise up inside of me. Yet I could not bear the thought...or perhaps my pride could not bear the thought of letting anyone know that I desperately wanted help. I saw how much pain I was already causing my parents and I could not for the life of me figure out how to make all of this go away. Pretending I was fine and that this was what I wanted helped me to deal with this.

I figured if they didn't see how much I was struggling or the intensity of the war inside, they wouldn't hurt as much. I couldn't allow them to get their hopes up when I was so quickly losing my grip and all hope. So I had to convince everyone, myself included, that this was what I wanted. On the other hand, my heart was already so numb at this point, God could have sent an angel down to confront me and I still would not have understood how dangerously close to the edge I was or how very capable God is to bring someone out of a struggle such as this, even as deep as I already was.

Eventually I began talking to girls at school, especially on nights where alcohol was involved. Mind you, I still had a boyfriend at this time. This life soon became comfortable, and turned into a cycle I could not seem to break free of, and though I knew I was hurting myself and others, I could not want to get out of it. I know that doesn't sound like it makes sense. But for the life of me, I wanted to want to go back to who and where I was. To this day, I'm not sure if it was pride or anger, or fear, or a combination of those and many other things, but I couldn't want to. And I desperately wanted to want to.

So the trouble is not with the law, for it is spiritual and good. The trouble is with me, for I am all too human, a slave to sin. I don't really understand myself, for I want to do what is right, but I don't do it. Instead, I do what I hate. But if I know that what I am doing is wrong, this shows that I agree that the law is good. So I am not the one doing wrong; it is sin living in me that does it. And I know that nothing good lives in me, that is, in my sinful nature. I want to do what is right, but I can't. I want to do what is good, but I don't. I don't want to do what is wrong, but I do it anyway. But if I do what I don't want to do, I am not really the one doing wrong; it is sin living in me that does it.

I have discovered this principle of life—that when I want to do what is right, I inevitably do what is wrong. I love God's law with all my heart. But there is another power within me that is at war with my mind. This power makes me a slave to the sin that is still within me. Oh, what a miserable person I am! Who will free me from this life that is dominated by sin and death? Thank God! The answer is in Jesus Christ our Lord. So you see how it is: In my mind I really want to obey God's law, but because of my sinful nature I am a slave to sin (Romans 7:14-25, NLT)

Sunday after Sunday I would go to the altar to try to pray because I could feel myself slipping away, the distance between myself and the God I once felt so close to, expanding at a rate I could not keep up with or seem to stop. I could no longer hear or feel the Holy Spirit, whereas I used to hear Him so clearly and feel His presence so strongly. There was one Sunday in particular, the last Sunday I sang in church. As we worshiped, I wondered to myself how many more songs were going to be played before I could sit down because though I could not hear or feel the Holy Spirit, I definitely felt uncomfortable in church.

Perhaps this was actually the Holy Spirit, and the discomfort from me fighting His touch. As I mouthed the words, my mind was everywhere else but on Him. One of the pastors took the microphone and said, "There is someone here who is singing these words but your heart is very far from Me. It would be better if you didn't sing at all". My mouth shut immediately. I couldn't sing worship songs after this. It was almost painful to even try.

Eventually I stopped going to the altar, stopped asking for prayer, stopped even trying to worship because I was angry that I was struggling. Angry, because I knew I could not live these very different lives. When my parents would go away for the weekend I would invite my friends over, many of whom had followed me when I was walking with Christ, and now were following as I ran further and further away. We would gather backpacks and take public transport to town, fill our bags with as much alcohol we could stuff in them, and head home to drink.

At 17 years old I was getting so drunk to the point where I would forget how to breathe or how to control my bladder. I also took up smoking around this time, which started as a "just when drinking" thing. I was still going to church on Sunday mornings, completely hungover, sweating vodka. I was eventually asked to step down from the leadership team, and though I was not surprised, I was hurt. I was offended. Church became a thing of the past and a source of immense pain.

Reading these journals has been very eye opening, because a few years into my rebellion I was fully convinced and telling anyone who asked that this was just "who I was" and that I was born this way. It had never even been a thought for me up until a very specific point in my life. In fact, remember my best friend's brother who I just knew I was in love with in Louisiana? We kept in touch via email after I moved away, and about a year or so after we moved he stopped talking to me. I didn't understand, but finally he wrote me a long letter telling me he loved me but that he was gay.

My heart shattered. I prayed and I prayed and I prayed for him. But I think I was more hurt than anything, feeling that I wasn't good enough. Though I was young, and it seems slightly pathetic, I was sure he was going to be my husband. I knew him for years, I never once considered that he was gay. Perhaps he had tendencies, but I didn't see it. All I saw was his joy, his love for Christ, and passion for worshipping. Those were the things I loved about him. And it broke my heart to see him turn away from God, from me. I didn't understand.

Many debate being born gay vs. becoming gay later in life. Homosexual desires may be so deeply rooted in someone's life that they genuinely believe they were born gay, as I eventually believed as well. Despite much research, there is no evidence that homosexuality is determined by any particular factor. In fact, more evidence shows that homosexuality may *not* be innate or unchangeable. I believe nature and nurture both play a role, in the sense that all of us are born into sin and with certain tendencies (many are issues such as pride and rebellion that manifest in different ways for different people). For me, it was pride and rebellion and a completely flawed sense of identity. I was introduced to homosexuality through playing soccer, which I was asked to give up. I entertained it because it allowed me to be prideful and rebellious and recreate my identity as I saw fit (I didn't realize at the time that this was what I was doing).

So, no, I was not born gay. This identity developed out of me not being obedient. Soccer became my life. How can I give up the only thing I'm good at? And the attention felt way too good. The value of my life, in my eyes, was determined by how much and who was showing me attention. And slowly but surely, I found myself in a place that all of a sudden felt too comfortable to walk away from. Feelings were too deep.

Not only was it just another thing I let define me, but it soon became the center point of my identity. I began pushing away any and everyone who tried to speak truth into my life, including my own family. I isolated myself, and I may have been having fun, but I never felt more lost and broken.

11/25/08:

Dear Jesus,

I'm such a screw up. I'm letting my family down I'm letting my friends down, I'm letting my pastors down and more importantly, I'm letting You down. You know all that's going on Jesus but for some reason I feel like I'm trying to hide when I don't write it all out. I'm not supposed to be seeing or talking to her anymore, but I have been. Finding any excuse to see her. I don't know why, Jesus. My mom said I need counseling and I'm beginning to agree. My youth pastor said he doesn't think I do because I know where and who I want to be so I just need to cut the crap and do it. I tried. I know why I like her…I've realized that I am attracted to girls who have some strength that I feel weak in, in my own life. I'm so insecure God. About who I am. I don't know who I am. I have lost my identity. And have resorted to finding it in other people who I think have strengths that I lack. I'm scared of so many things. I don't think I'm a great singer. I don't think I'm good enough in soccer. I'm a push-over. But I want to be confident, so I look for that strength in others and not in You. And the thing is, they probably are just as insecure as I am. Jesus…I know you have blessed us all with talents…please help me to see my worth in You! Help me to find my identity in You, Father. Only You. I need You so badly right now. I'm way off track. My Mimi doesn't even think I'm a Christian anymore. She preached to me tonight. I keep being rude to my mom. I'm sorry, Jesus. When I try to talk to her about it she cries. I miss my dad.

I want to feel on fire for You like I used to. I want to be on fire for You again. I NEED YOU, Jesus…how do I get out of this pit I've thrown myself into? I want to find my strength in You. Please forgive me, yet again, for falling back into this Jesus. I'm tired of messing up but this probably won't be the last time…so please forgive me for then too. You are all I need. You are more than enough. Help me to see that Jesus. I love you. Please help her to see that I want out, and please help her to want out too. Give me strength not to like her anymore Jesus, please.

If you can relate, whether a little or completely, even if it is not with this particular struggle, please know that if you simply come, believing that He is, His sovereignty will supersede all of your doubt. This has nothing to do with your strength or ability and everything to do with His love and victory. His blood is enough to break every chain.

Therefore He is able also to save to the uttermost (completely, perfectly, finally, and for all time and eternity) those who come to God through Him, since He is always living to make petition to God and intercede with Him and intervene for them (Hebrews 7:25, AMP).

Lean on, trust in, and be confident in the Lord with all your heart and mind and do not rely on your own insight or understanding. In all your ways know, recognize, and acknowledge Him, and He will direct and make straight and plain your paths (Proverbs 3:5-6 AMP).

Keep reading…

CHAPTER 5: RUNNING OUT OF HIDING

"Will it ever end?!? I'm a disaster!! HELP ME!! I AM NOT A LESBIAN Jesus help me"

December of 2008 was the last time I wrote in my journal for many years. Journaling was always my line of communication with God. When I didn't write, it was probably because, though I know He sees and knows all, I felt guilty and was trying to hide. After this entry it was because I was tired of falling, tired of trying to focus on all the things I shouldn't do, tired of trying in my own strength to get myself out of this. So, because we serve a God who is not limited in the way He communicates with us, I still felt Him tugging on my heart. Which only meant I had to increase the frequency and intensity of my studying, but also of my drinking, smoking and partying whenever and wherever possible in order to block Him out and maintain the numbness I despised but desperately needed in order to continue living as I pleased.

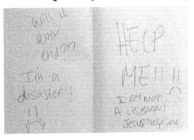

Distractions.

I needed at all times to be distracted. So distracted that soccer was becoming less and less of a priority, perhaps, in part, because it no longer felt so great to run nonstop for 90 minutes after having stayed up the night before doing who knows what.

4/19/08:
Let Me In
Father, where are You?
I'm right beside you.
Why have You left me?
I will not leave you...
Why can't I feel You?
Child, you can hear Me.
Why won't You hold me?
I would if you'd let Me.
Why won't you let Me in to heal your broken heart?
Don't you know it breaks Mine to see you fall apart?
How can you turn away after all I've brought you through?
I formed you in the womb. The love of My life is you.
Love...let Me in, let Me in.
Just let Me hold you, It's all gonna be okay.
Let me wash you clean with My healing grace
Give Me your tomorrow, I'll get you through today
Beloved, I long for you and in My arms you'll stay.
Jesus, please hold me. I would if you'd let me...in.

8/10/08:
Truth
I'm tired of walking this dark road
And I can't do it on my own
I'm at the point of desperation

Crying out in my frustration
Why can't I feel you?
Does that mean You are not there?
And I can't hear Your voice
Does that mean You do not care?

Let me speak some truth over this situation.
Let me speak some truth over this situation.
Let me speak some truth over you.
Yes, I can hear you.
And yes, I care.
I will not leave you
I've always been there
I am Your Father
I am Your Savior
I am your deliverer and redeemer
I am I AM.

Above are two songs I wrote, and tried to throw away. Thankfully, my sisters found and saved them, because I now see that even in this place, He was trying to draw me in. And I was seeking. Until I gave up the fight. However, it is so comforting to know that even when we give up on ourselves, when we give up on Him, He never gives up the fight. Over the next few years, I did whatever I wanted (whatever I could get away with while still living with, and to some very limited extent, obeying my parents).

Lying became second nature to me very quickly, because that was the only way I could get what I wanted. I manipulated and guilt tripped and blatantly lied about many things, usually in order to see whoever I was talking to at the time. I had a few boyfriends in the beginning, but mostly to keep my parents' suspicion and concern at bay. Eventually, I didn't even care who knew or what they thought. Anyone who had something to say about my choices was closed minded and hateful and I was quick to make sure they knew it.

I cannot remember a specific time that I sat down and "came out" to my family, per say, but I didn't have to. They saw my Facebook. I avoided them so I would not have to talk about it. I despised long car rides with my mom and avoided them at all costs, because she would always find a way to bring it up. One time, on the way to Nelspruit, South Africa, where we went often for doctor's appointments, we got into an argument about her worship music, which I could not stand listening to.

This had become a common complaint of mine, and usually led to a heated argument over my lifestyle choices. I told her I could not help it, that I had tried, and that she was going to have to accept me for who I was. She began to cry, and through sobs asked me what she had done wrong. It broke my heart. But I was way too far in. My dad didn't say much to me about it, I don't know if it was because he wasn't sure what to say, or if he just realized earlier than my mom that it was entirely out of his hands.

In 2009 I started talking to someone that was introduced to me by a friend at school who observed that my family situation and "coming out" had taken quite the toll on me. She thought it would be helpful to speak with her cousin, who a few years earlier had gone through something similar. She and I initially only spoke via Facebook and Mxit a few days a week. A few days a week turned to every morning and every night before bed. Soon, every second of every day. I never seemed to have enough money on my phone (air-time) anymore because I was constantly talking to her.

She lived in South Africa and for the first year of our relationship she was still in med school and could not come see me very often. The first time she came to Swaziland to see me in person, my ex boy-friend offered to take me to meet her as I had no transportation. I was so nervous to meet her in person he had to lift me out of the car and push me into the building. This relationship, though mostly long distance, was the deepest, most intimate relationship I have ever experienced.

In the beginning of our relationship I was a little scared of how quickly my life had turned in this direction and I almost ended it at one point because of this. It was as if my soul's cry, very briefly, rose to the point I could hear and feel, and the depth of the pain as I continued to use all of my strength to completely push God out of my life was almost too much to bear. It nearly broke her heart. That day I had a soccer game a few hours' drive away from home, and had no airtime on my phone to call her. I cried the whole way there and back and as soon as I was able to get airtime, called and frantically apologized.

I remember threatening to sit in the middle of a busy road in the freezing cold if she wouldn't forgive me and give me another chance (I would have if there were busy roads in Swaziland in the middle of the night). She became my lifeline. My life. I loved her so much that though I still felt God tugging on my heart, I was ready to completely turn my back and ignore Him if it meant I got to keep her. Our relationship quickly got to the point where I could not imagine a day without her. The more I ran from God, the more desperately I needed her love.

In order to see her, before my parents knew about our relationship, I lied and said I wanted to go visit a doctor friend in SA in order to see if I wanted to be a doctor. I had no intention of ever becoming a doctor. She would take a bus to see me occasionally on weekends and with my parents believing I was staying with a friend at school, I would meet her at a guest house or hotel. Once my parents began to catch on to my lies and what was really going on we had to learn to be more discreet. I learned how to play basketball and made the team that would travel to Johannesburg for a weekend tournament just so that I would be closer to her. She flew to Johannesburg to see me for 1 hour and then flew back to where she lived.

She would have done anything for me, and I was willing to risk it all to prove my love for her. I had a few jaw surgeries, the last one leaving half of my face paralyzed for 6 months, and she tried to come see me in the hospital. My mom wouldn't let her visit me, though she had gotten off of a 36 hour shift and spent a lot of money to take a plane to where I was. I was furious. I felt like she was being irrational. Life was so unfair. I cried and cursed her and my sisters as they cried too because they could see I was in pain, and though I didn't enjoy hurting them, I was so deeply doing just that.

Towards the end of my time in Swaziland, while in my second year of IB, I stole money from my parents, took my passport, lied and said I was staying at school to study for midterm exams, and hopped on a bus, which was pulling a trailer full of chickens, for 10 hours to Durban, South Africa. My girlfriend, by the way, did not condone this, nor did she know I was doing this until I was already on my way there. My parents have never been (despite my teenage assumptions) dumb and quickly found out where I was, when my mom had this sudden feeling she should look at our passports. And I, being the very intelligent person that I am, turned on my phone once in South Africa so that when she called my South African number to see if by some chance this nightmare was real, it rang. That phone call did not go very well.

I knew I had already broken their hearts but now it felt as if I was twisting the knife. And while I sat there dumbfounded, I wondered how I was going to enjoy the remainder of my getaway when I had no idea what would be waiting for me once I got home. While on Facebook that very day, I saw a picture my sister had posted of her and my mom at lunch. My mom's eyes were so swollen and her smile so weary. The bus ride home to Swaziland was the longest journey of my life. I contemplated running away for good. I planned out what I would do if my parents did not pick me up once I got back to Swaziland, if they kicked me out.

My dad picked me up. Once home, they sat me down in the living room across from them. My mom had no more tears to cry, nor words to say. My dad began to cry. And through his tears, told me they had given up. I was free to do whatever I wanted. They had already bought my one-way ticket to the United States, as we were going back that winter once I graduated and the plan was that I would be staying there for college. It was my decision if I got on the plane with them or not, but they no longer cared what I did.

This was the response I had wanted from them for years, wasn't it? I was free! This didn't feel like freedom. I felt desperately trapped. Part of me just wanted to stay behind and go live with my girlfriend in South Africa and cut ties with everyone else. The thought of moving even farther away from her was incredibly painful. But I knew I had to go to the States as I had just spent 2 extremely grueling years completing the IB program and was sure to be offered at least a partial scholarship to nursing school. My girlfriend offered to send me to school if I stayed there, but I had seen how nurses in Swaziland and South Africa were treated and I had no desire to be a doctor. I knew I had to go to the States.

And though I felt more distant from my family than ever, my heart longed to be close to them. I felt safe with them. Despite all that had happened, they were still my family, and I knew they loved me immensely. In order to not have to deal with these very intense and conflicting emotions, I began avoiding my family altogether. Living in a room separate from the main house made this a little easier. For the most part, my siblings and I stopped talking. My brother completely cut me off. They began confiding in Lizzy and considering her to be the big sister I could no longer be.

The principal of my school (who was my girlfriend's uncle) met with my parents once the situation had become so tense and he offered to allow me to live on campus for free for my last term, just to be able to focus on exams. Not knowing what else to do, they agreed. The distance helped us all to keep our calm throughout my last few months in Swaziland. I felt persecuted and so alone, all the while knowing I had somehow put myself in this situation. I was so distraught during these last few months that I lost quite a bit of weight and hair. I was terrified of leaving.

I felt my girlfriend pulling away because she was terrified too. Somehow I managed to convince her that I was not going to move away and forget about her. I promised her I would return and we would get married. And live happily ever after. And I believed this with all of my heart. The start of this new chapter felt like the end of the world. My heart felt like it was being ripped in half. But I had to believe so that she would believe. My biggest fear was that she would let the fear and sadness of me leaving cause her to end our relationship.

CHAPTER 6: HOME OF THE FREE

I moved back to the United States in 2010 to live with my Mimi in Baton Rouge, completed a certified nursing assistant (CNA) program and began working at Sunrise Senior Living as a nursing assistant. Relieved to have distance between my family and I so I wasn't constantly aware of the tension, I was enjoying my freedom as a working adult in the USA. However, it took me a while to adjust to the fast pace. Everyone always seemed to be in a hurry and there were so many people everywhere! I had very much so come to love and appreciate the slow paced, relaxed atmosphere in Swaziland.

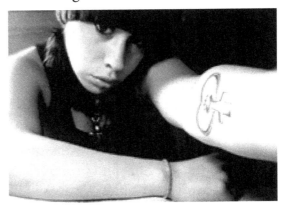

I made some friends in Baton Rouge and would sometimes go out partying or drinking, always trying to make sure I was home, still awake and sober enough to talk to my girlfriend when she woke up (she was either 6 or 7 hours ahead of me depending on what time of the year it was and which time zone I was in). Being so far away and with the time difference, our relationship was very strained and at times left both of us feeling depressed. However, I was adjusting to a whole new life and was more distracted than she was, so she often felt like I had forgotten about her. I got a tattoo on my back, my first tattoo, of our favorite quote and her initials, just so she would know how sure I was of my love for her.

I moved to Baltimore and began nursing school in 2011, and would travel back to South Africa and Swaziland on summer breaks to visit my then, fiancé, and family. These summers were difficult because my parents obviously wanted me to spend more time with them, but I wanted to be in South Africa. And my parents loved me enough to respect that, though it hurt them. It was my hope and dream that my parents would give their stamp of approval. To my great surprise, excitement, and complete terror, they actually said yes when I asked if she could come to the house for tea and games one day.

She was terrified. I was terrified. My brother locked himself in his room. My dad was friendly, said hi, and went about his business. My youngest sister was the only sibling who made an appearance and she, my mom, my girlfriend, and I played spades over tea and brownies. This meant so much to me. At the time, I thought I was on my way to obtaining their approval; inviting them to our future wedding became a tiny bit less scary. Now, I see how they were just desperately trying not to push me away, trying to love me, not by necessarily approving, but loving me where I was at, despite how they felt.

I come from a family that is extremely Christian and conservative. My parents are missionaries in southern Africa. I am the oldest daughter. I used to be the big sister they all looked up to. Two years ago I came out, and my life has never been the same. I do not regret my decision to tell my family and finally be honest with myself. I am now happy and comfortable with who I am, and I have an amazing girlfriend in South Africa, whom I love more than life. However, I wish I still had the relationships with my siblings that I used to. I wish my parents accepted me for who I am. I wish me being a lesbian wasn't the "unspoken" in our house. I wish I didn't feel like I have to try so hard to make them proud to make up for the disappointment I caused them. I would love to be able to use what I learn in this class to help girls who have been through similar situations as I have, who struggle with who they are because others do not accept them. (Women's Studies Journal- February 1st, 2012)

A few months after this journal entry, I ruined my relationship. I was getting attention at school, too caught up in soccer, and had made some new, older friends outside of school as well. I cheated. This led to a string of empty flings and short-term relationships where I was either 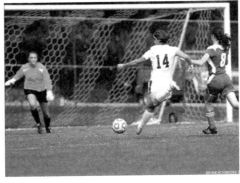 left broken hearted, or hurt someone else, each one leaving me feeling more empty than before. All the while I was trying to get my ex in South Africa to forgive and take me back because I felt I had messed up the best thing that had ever happened to me. In all of my relationships I felt that I was searching for what I had with her, and I hated myself for breaking her trust, for breaking her heart.

CHAPTER 7: TOO MUCH AND NEVER ENOUGH

I became vice-president of my campus LGBT group and became involved in LGBT activism and decided I was also going to be a feminist. So, naturally, I had to get tattoos all over my body to display these things in which I stood for, and in which my identity was found. You see, when I was deciding on a university, it was between Maryland and Iowa. I chose to come to Maryland, because I knew that the Baltimore, DC area was a hot-spot for LGBT activism. I wanted to stand for something, to fight for something, and this was my cause.

I had the phrase "λove what you λove" tattooed across my ribs after researching the Greek lambda symbol (λ), which is equivalent to the English letter "L". This symbol was officially declared the international symbol for gay and lesbian rights by the International Gay Rights Congress in Edinburgh, Scotland in 1974. I had the feminist symbol tattooed on my forearm. I became extremely anti-men, which I realize is not the point of feminism for many, but the idea of women's rights and equality with men stirred up an anger in me that extended far beyond rights and equality. The idea of any man being above or controlling me angered me to the point of tears. Looking back, I think this had a lot to do with my anger and rebellion towards God. I had a tattoo designed of the Greek mother goddess, Gaia, and would have a full body tattoo now if I had not been a poor college student and could afford it.

Instead of Gaia, I had a quote tattooed across my chest from a poem by my favorite LGBT activist and spoken word poet, Andrea Gibson, Glider Plane: "This heart is my Sunday best". When I was little my Mimi used to dress us up in matching dresses she and my PawPaw would get us on their trips to the mountains. She used to tell us we had to wear our Sunday best to worship Jesus, so yes, I HAD to wear the itchy, poofy dress, despite my strong disapproval. Getting this tattooed across my chest was my way of saying to those who refused to accept me that this is my best. This is me. This is all I have to offer, so stop expecting and praying for something, someone else.

Throughout my time in college, I attended events such as Bmore Proud where we met up with other LGBT college students and professionals to celebrate ourselves and discuss issues such as discrimination, safe sex, and expressing ourselves in music, poetry, and drag. I also volunteered and participated in a NOH8 photoshoot, further expressing my passion for this cause.

This past weekend was Bmore Proud at UMBC. To be quite honest, I feel like a new person. What I learned there and the feeling of being part of a community where we, as the LGBTQIA community are not only accepted, but loved, encouraged, in-

spired, and motivated was one of the best experiences in my life thus far. I think it is so important for youth and young adults to attend events such as Bmore Proud, so that they can be inspired to make a difference, whether big or small, in our community. This is important so we can fight for rights to be able to do all of the things we may not be able to do yet. There is progress, though, as we saw last week with the passing of the Same Sex Marriage Bill. However, there is still so much more to do, and I am so excited to do whatever I can to make a difference. (Women's Studies Class Journal 3/21/12)

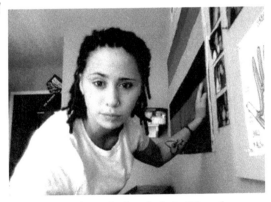

During all of this time I could not figure out whether I wanted to be more "dominant" or "feminine". I was asked to further label myself as a "fem", a "stud", or many different labels in between. I decided I didn't like the labels, so I would adapt to whoever I was dating at the time. But if push came to shove and you asked me enough times, I would tell you I was a "stem"- safely in the middle. If the person was more feminine, I would take on the masculine or dominant role (or try to) and if they were more dominant, I would try to be more feminine. A source of much heartache, this usually didn't work, because I was always too much something and not enough something else. When trying to be something you are not, there is always going to be a "too", because it is in your own strength and not according to His plan for your life.

Truthfully, dressing up like a boy and taking on that role

became most comfortable because I felt more guarded in this identity. It made me feel tough. There were times when I would walk past another girl dressed in a similar manner that I thought was cute and I would wish in that moment that I was dressed more "girly", but then feel crushed wondering if I even looked good as a girl anymore, if she would have noticed me anyways. I had similar thoughts when I saw guy I thought was cute, but I quickly reminded myself that I was anti-men and could not allow such thoughts. My femininity had been wounded, and is something that God is still restoring, reminding me that I am beautifully feminine, just the way He made me.

For you formed my inward parts; you knitted me together in my mother's womb. I praise you, for I am fearfully and wonderfully made. Wonderful are your works; my soul knows it very well. My frame was not hidden from you, when I was being made in secret, intricately woven in the depths of the earth. Your eyes saw my unformed substance; in your book were written, every one of them, the days that were formed for me, when as yet there was none of them. How precious to me are your thoughts, O God! How vast is the sum of them! (Psalm 139:13-17, NKJV)

CHAPTER 8: IF YOU ARE NOT REAL

As I attended a Catholic university, I had to take religious studies as one of my classes. I was a little nervous about this, because at this point I had become anti anything and everything pertaining to God, in any way, shape or form. I stopped playing my guitar, because through all of this, every time I picked up my guitar to play, the only songs that would come to mind were worship songs. To my great relief, the professor of this religious studies class basically told us all that the Bible could not be taken literally in many instances, and that most was open to interpretation. When I wrote my final paper on me being the black sheep of my family because I was gay, comparing it to the story of the Prodigal Son, I got an A, and an encouraging word from my professor.

Ever since I came out to my family, I have constantly felt like they look at me with pity and hope that I will one day all of the sudden change. I was kicked out of the church leadership team, and also the worship team when they found out I was a lesbian. Every opportunity they got, my mom or one of my younger siblings would preach to me about how I need to "return to God". I honestly would feel like when the prodigal son was brought up in church or conversation, my family would look at me, because in their eyes, I am just like the prodigal son. I know they pray continuously for me to recognize that what I am doing is wrong (in their eyes) and to return to the Father. They do not understand that I never left Him. I just felt like I had no place belonging to Him anymore, so I pushed away. I did start to do things that probably were not smart or right, and they would have been right to compare me to the prodigal son then, but not when it comes to who I love. After reading this parable and looking into it in depth, I can, to a small extent, relate my family to the Pharisees in that they made me feel (not intentionally) that I had no place in the Kingdom of God. This is why this passage means so much to me, because the father was willing to do anything to mend the broken relationships and show compassion to his hurting son, even if it meant going against all cultural and religious norms. Sometimes, I wish my family would do the same. When we first were told about this exegesis, I saw the parable of the prodigal son and immediately crossed it off the list, because it made me mad to think about all that was associated with it in my mind. Writing this exegesis has made me realize that God is not the One who changed. He has always been the same loving, compassionate, caring Father I always knew Him to be, and I will no longer let anyone change that for me. Many Christians unknowingly act like the Pharisees and judge when they have no place to. If people could take away one thing from this parable, I think it should be to try and learn from the father, because you never know how you could impact or touch someone's life by showing them unconditional compassion just as the father showed his son, and how God showed us by giving us His only son to die for us. (Exegesis: Parable of the Ever Joyous Father, November 13, 2012)

At this point, I was feeling more set in my identity and had received the affirmation I thought I was yearning for at school, from professors I respected (even religious professors). I had felt God's call on my life from a young age and my spirit longed for Him. Church was something that I missed, as it had been a place of comfort and community for most of my life. I decided I wanted to try to go back to church, so I would just have to find a church with a rainbow flag on the outside, as I now knew there were many who preached that it was okay to be gay and Christian. I attended a Unitarian Universalist church, where we sang hymns, Buddhist chants, and read poetry.

It was a nice gathering of a very diverse and friendly group of people, but I could not worship. The words wouldn't come out. It felt like I was trying to put on a show for God, and having experienced His presence so strongly through worship in my past, my spirit would not allow me to mock Him by singing words I didn't understand or mean, and to a god or gods that were not Him. Sin cannot find an audience with God. Even at this time, I knew this. Just because I was now more comfortable with myself, did not mean the relationship had been restored. And I dared not set foot in a church where I knew I would feel the Holy Spirit's conviction.

Eventually, I decided I would just have to believe there wasn't a God, that this would be so much easier. When I mentioned this to one of my friends, she excitedly had me watch a documentary with her called Zeitgeist, where many different topics were discussed, one being that Christianity is a myth. The only problem was that the thought of this, when I truly thought about it, almost had me crash my car into a tree on my drive home, because the thought of there not being a God was more painful than anything I ever went through or imagined. I realized that if this were the case, there was absolutely no purpose in existing. None. At all.

Thankfully, even in this place of darkness and confusion, despite my efforts to try and justify my actions and my feelings by convincing myself God was not real, I could not bring myself to do this. You cannot un-know Christ. And the more I tried, the less everything made sense and the more I felt I was losing my mind. I had already experienced too much of Him to even begin to discount Him. Which only made living this lifestyle so much harder. He was so obvious. I saw Him in, through, and despite everything. And in this moment of despair, my sister sent me a link to the song "Oceans" by Hillsong United. And as I drove aimlessly through the city, trying to see through tear-filled eyes, completely submerged in the words to this song, His presence flooded my heart and soul and I knew I could never deny Him.

They know the truth about God because he has made it obvious to them. For ever since the world was created, people have seen the earth and sky. Through everything God made, they can clearly see his invisible qualities—his eternal power and divine nature. So they have no excuse for not knowing God. Yes, they knew God, but they wouldn't worship him as God or even give him thanks. And they began to think up foolish ideas of what God was like. As a result, their minds became dark and confused. Claiming to be wise, they instead became utter fools. And instead of worshiping the glorious, ever-living God, they worshiped idols made to look like mere people and birds and animals and reptiles (Romans 1:19-23, NLT).

However, I wasn't ready to deny myself, either. It is important to understand that there is a distinction between relationship with Jesus and relationship with church or with religion. The answer to the question, *"Who do you say that I am?" (Matthew 16:15)* becomes key in deciphering which it is you have or seek. Like Peter, I had already answered this question in my heart many years prior.

Simon Peter answered, "You are the Messiah, the Son of the living God. "Jesus replied, "You are blessed, Simon son of John, because my Father in heaven has revealed this to you. You did not learn this from any human being (Matthew 16:16-17, NLT).

In my seeking a church and in all of the times I found myself in a church, particularly the ones that did speak truth and Jesus, my spirit would stir at the mention of His Name. I did not like this stirring- which is why I tried to avoid this. My spirit longed for Him, and I longed for the familiarity of the relationship to church, to a church family, without the threat of conviction or correction. I thought I was seeking God, but in truth I was seeking for my identity to be confirmed by the God I knew in my heart of hearts would never tell me what I wanted to hear or condone the way I was living or the person I was becoming. I wanted both. I wanted to hold on to my identity, my life, my sin, and to have Him too. It didn't work out very well, but I wasn't ready to make the sacrifice and surrender. I wasn't ready to choose Him.

Journal- May 2013
The very foundations on which I stood stand shaking trembling beneath me and I am uncertain I know how to walk forward without them crumbling and I, crashing, hardly able to see straight through the tears I reach out hands open grasping anything solid that might not slip through the spaces between my fingers...
We all need something, someone to believe in and when your

whole life has been centered on this one thing...

What if it is not real?

I would not know where to go from there. Do I blindly believe and deny the facts or do I push aside something that was my world my whole life and accept that in our need of something more to believe in all that we lived for was created in a beautiful story to bring hope because we could not accept that there was nothing.

I cannot accept that there is nothing. Nothing is more difficult to believe than something and I know what I feel though I cannot put it into words because at this very moment my heart is shattered and I am trying to put the pieces back together.

This puzzle cannot be solved. This puzzle has too many pieces.

Maybe there is so much more than all that I ever believed. Maybe that was just one corner of the puzzle and in order for it to make sense I must step back and try to take in the whole.

I fear the entirety of it may be too much for my mind to comprehend, for my heart to bear...

But my soul...my soul takes flight because it knows that me realizing there is more to the puzzle is already one step closer to getting there.

There may be relative and somewhere I never find, some things may never make sense.

I accept this, find my footing, take a deep breath, and remember that this journey is not mine.

CHAPTER 9: HE SIMPLY SAID, "GUARD YOUR HEART"

I returned home to Swaziland in the summer of 2013 with two of my best friends from school, as we had been awarded a grant to conduct a Davis Peace Project. We would be working with a group of ladies in Section 19, which is one of the rural communities my parents work in. These ladies already had a sewing project up and running 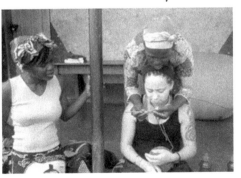 and had learned to sew the most beautiful bags, which my parents help them sell in order to bring money back into their community. We decided that we would teach them to crochet, so we flew to Swaziland with suitcases full of yarn, as they both tried to teach me to crochet on the way there. To this day I still do not know how to crochet; the kids distracted me and I was completely useless except to untangle the yarn and make everyone sandwiches.

My mom has become very close to these women through discipleship over the past few years- they have Bible studies, worship and pray together. I recently found out that before we arrived in Swaziland, my mom had warned the ladies that I may look and act differently than they remember. She told

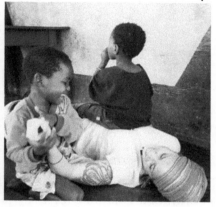

them a little of what had been going on and asked them to help her pray for me. I was shocked that they did not say more to me about my 11 tattoos or 18 piercings, that I made no attempts, whatsoever, to hide, even though my parents asked me to, out of respect for their culture. The ladies caught on to crocheting so quickly that they ended up trying to teach me to crochet! This became their unified mission- but, like I said, the kids distracted me and completely stole my heart and attention.

While there, my mom asked me to go to church with them, but I refused every time, and I could tell it hurt her heart. God made it clear to her during this time I was back home, as she was able to see firsthand how much I had changed, how far I had strayed, that it would be nothing that she did that would bring me back. She had to surrender and trust His heart. One day, I had a major fallout with my siblings about the amount of alcohol I was consuming and who I was bringing into the house.

My brother confronted me and I did not take it very well. It ended with both of my sisters standing up for my brother as I cursed him out, the three of them locking themselves in my brother's room, all of us crying, and me sobbing on the back porch. Hurt. Scared. Empty. And so angry at myself for the hateful words that I never in a million years thought would come out of my mouth, and towards one of the people I love most in this world, my own brother. When my parents returned, my dad took me, in all of my crying glory, to a coffee shop, simply to talk to me. I sobbed about what had just happened and how I always felt judged by everyone. I sobbed about the fact that my heart had been broken so many times recently and none of them ever even asked how my personal life was or how my heart was. He then told me to tell him everything.

Completely shocked, I did not hesitate, and I told all. I told him about the girls I had met and dated from the dating website, OkCupid. How one I really liked, took me on a date and then cut me off, only to apologize one year later, take me on another date, get my hopes up, and realize "oh, she's still the same person who 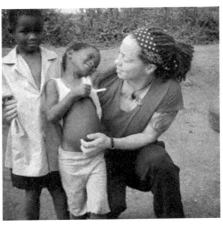 wasn't what I was looking for last year" and cut me off again. I told him about the one who said she liked me but knew she would break my heart so she did not want to commit, which, of course, broke my heart.

I told him about every person I liked who I was either too young for, too sensitive, too innocent, too gullible. I told him about the girlfriend who tried to choke me after I broke up with her. I told him about all the people I had hurt, who also weren't what I was looking for, therefore making me no better than any of the ones who hurt me. How I felt like I was looking for my ex in all of them. How painful it was to be back in Swaziland, where everything reminded me of her. He listened attentively to my drama, and then left me with three words I had heard before, but that came to mind very often over the next few years after this coffee date. He simply told me to guard my heart. Sounds easy, right? It sounded completely ridiculous to me in this very moment. It left me bewildered, because at this time I was realizing I didn't feel like I had any heart left to protect.

While in Swaziland, I left my car with a girl I really liked. This was the person who told me she liked me but was afraid of hurting me. I hoped that in me allowing her to use my car, since she did not have one, (which was not a very wise thing to do looking back) would somehow win her over. However, it was mid-trip when she began ignoring me that I wished with all my heart I could call my grandparents and have them go get my car. But, I then remembered that I had lied to them about where my car was, because when I suggested lending it to someone, they confirmed what I already knew but disregarded- not a wise decision.

Upon returning to Baltimore and regaining custody of Pegasus (my white 2005 Pontiac Grand Am that overheated if the heat was not on full blast at all times), I returned to OkCupid. Within a few weeks, I began dating someone I met online. This relationship was particularly difficult, because at this point I had gotten used to dressing as a tom-boy, sometimes in full boy attire, and she did not approve of this at all. She was the "dominant" one and I was supposed to dress and act like a lady. In a sense, I suppose I had deceived her because I did dress more feminine on our first few dates. I tried to explain that I was both and I didn't understand what the big deal was. We had many fights over this topic, and I finally began allowing her to pick and buy my outfits.

A poor college student, who used most of her money eating out and on alcohol, I needed more money. So I did what anyone does when they need more money. I began the process of "donating" my eggs. Which involved a few months of abstaining from alcohol and all forms of smoking, followed by 6 months of bloodwork, self-injecting hormones and sometimes daily 6am checkups at the fertility clinic. Thankfully, my mom was in town when I had the surgery to harvest the eggs, because I was a mess. It's already hard enough being a hormonal female (particularly once a month).

Add extra hormones, constant bloating, weight gain, and a warning that quick movement, running, or jumping could twist the follicles leading to pelvic inflammatory disease, and you have a HOT mess. I survived. And because I am smart, I used a good majority of the money to adopt my girlfriend and I a child (a toy poodle), which I was extremely allergic to. Our fighting worsened and became more often- the poodle was not helping the situation, as I had hoped. We broke up. She kept the poodle.

I Can Go On- 2013
Ten years ago if you would have shown me my future, I would have undoubtedly laughed…we're moving to Africa? Us? yeah right…Swaziland is NOT a real place.
We moved to Africa.
Eight years ago if you would have told me I was going to finally come out the closet and break my family's heart, I would have been shocked. I'm not gay…I'm a Christian!
I exploded out that damn closet.
Five years ago if you would have told me I was about to meet my future fiancé, I would have…believed you, and been ecstatic, because indeed, even at 17 I was already a hopeless romantic.
I met her and fell madly in love.

Three years ago if you would have told me this love was not going to last forever, I would not have even allowed you to finish your sentence. We were beautiful. We were all there was.

We did not make forever.

A year ago if you would have told me I would have so many heartbreaks, so many failed love affairs, so many emotions threatening to drown me daily, confused, lonely, wandering... waiting. broken, hopeful, broken again...searching. stars hidden. hope fallen. blood boiling...butterflies f* them...I hate butterflies. maybe she's the one. that went badly. this hurts is it supposed to hurt? tomorrow will be better. not again...

I am still waiting.

Still

Waiting...

We do not know what the future holds. All I have is here and now and I am hopeful that in ten years when I look back and rewrite this, it will go something like this:

Ten years ago I was broken, empty, lost, hurting, confused...and if you would have told me I'd be happy, in love, loved, treasured, butterflies? I love butterflies...

I would have smiled, I am smiling. Because in the midst of this whirlwind I find peace knowing that life takes some pretty incredible, unexpected turns...like the words on this page...

Not even I know what direction they will take...but the only thing that matters is that they keep going. They keep going until I decided to end the sentence and set my pencil down.

They keep going until my hand can write no more, until I am too tired and weak to go on, and I have a lot of strength left.

I can go on...

CHAPTER 10: NOW THAT I'VE GOT YOUR ATTENTION

My sister moved to the United States in 2013, and I had reached a breaking point. My heart was hurting from the last few failed relationships I had been in. I had taken up bartending on a dinner cruise-ship at the Inner Harbor. Some of the midday cruises, particularly if they were children's parties, were slow, which meant that the bartenders didn't really do much except make smoothies and Shirley Temples. This left much time for chit-chat and usually we worked in pairs. One of the other bartenders I worked with frequently on these day cruises shared with me that she was a Christian. I opened up to her and explained my life story, and was not at all judged or made to feel like any less of a person or child of God (I suppose I looked for this when someone said they were a Christian, though I suppose in part it was actually my own convictions). She invited me to visit her church, where I was told about a women's conference they would be having in February of that year.

My sister was living in Pennsylvania, working on her CNA license, and struggling to adjust to being back in the States after having just spent the last year traveling the world with

Youth with a Mission (YWAM). I invited her to go to the conference with me, as I thought it would be good for both of us to get away and be able to spend time together. I was also desperately hoping for something. A sign. A word. A touch. Anything. We met in Gettysburg, Pennsylvania for a weekend full of fellowship and worship. I felt God so strongly throughout this weekend.

During one of the breaks in between sessions, my sister introduced me to former lesbian and spoken word artist, Jackie Hill, now Jackie Hill Perry. Well, on YouTube, anyways. She showed me the piece she wrote called My Life as a Stud, where Jackie speaks about her experiences living in the homosexual lifestyle and how God called her out. She then showed me the video where Jackie's (now) husband, Preston, performed a spoken word piece asking her to marry him. Both touched my heart deeply and I found such hope in her testimony. God pursued her heart as I knew He had been pursuing mine, and then once she returned, showered love on her like she had never experienced it before, just because that is how much He loves His daughter. I went back to school after this weekend feeling renewed, but deathly afraid. The following passage was a journal entry after going for a run the day I returned from the retreat.

Listen- February 2014

Just as I was about to turn the last corner that signified the end of my run, a still small voice whispered, "Keep going, I have so much to show you."

He led me down a small street I had never noticed. It was quiet. Peaceful. I felt His love in the shiver that radiated through my body. The nearness of Him almost made me forget I was running.

The road suddenly came to an end and I was on the main road once more. Such an abrupt change. Cars flying by. People. Running. Walking. Too close. My heart began to race, my lungs tried to keep up, and I was suddenly aware that my legs were indeed tired...I nearly stopped...

But the whisper..." Keep going My child. Keep going." I closed my eyes for a brief second and asked Him to steady my heart. I once more reached the place where my run was to come to an end...but I still felt my journey to be incomplete.

I ran past a graveyard and turned around, only noticing it in my second passing. Something overcame me. My heart, lungs, and legs stopped and as I stood there staring at the tombstones, a song came to mind...and I finally understood.

"No guilt in life, no fear in death- this is the power of Christ in me. From life's first cry to final breath, Jesus commands my destiny. No power of hell, no scheme of man, can ever pluck me from His hand. Till He returns or calls me home, here in the power of Christ, I'll stand."

This journey will not always be comfortable and peaceful. You will not always feel Me or hear Me through the chaos and confusion. There will be distractions. But through all of this, you are Mine. I command your destiny, not you. I knew who you would be before you were even a thought, I knew all of the twists and turns and I have GREAT plans for your life. Your purpose is not yet complete. We have only just begun. Your identity is in Me, alone.

And I. Will. Not. Let. You. Go.

Keep going. I have so much to show you...now that I've got your attention.

While at the retreat, a lady prayed for me, someone, who, to this day is a very special friend. I felt and heard Him telling me it was time to stop running away from Him and to start journeying with Him, but I was not yet ready to truly listen. I returned to school feeling refreshed, but I didn't seek fellowship. I didn't get plugged in at church. I wasn't ready to make any real changes and trying with all my (key-word 'my') might to NOT do things or talk to certain people only made me want to do them more. I was frustrated by my lack of faith and my inability to pull myself together. So, I fell back in, ten times deeper than I had been before. You see, when we only focus on all of the things we shouldn't be doing rather than the new life we have in Christ, the new life He promises us in all of its fullness, we are trying to live solely by the law and not through His grace.

So, my dear brothers and sisters, this is the point: You died to the power of the law when you died with Christ. And now you are united with the one who was raised from the dead. As a result, we can produce a harvest of good deeds for God. When we were controlled by our old nature, sinful desires were at work within us, and the law aroused these evil desires that produced a harvest of sinful deeds, resulting in death. But now we have been released from the law, for we died to it and are no longer captive to its power. Now we can serve God, not in the old way of obeying the letter of the law, but in the new way of living in the Spirit. Well then, am I suggesting that the law of God is sinful? Of course not! In fact, it was the law that showed me my sin. I would never have known that coveting is wrong if the law had not said, "You must not covet." But sin used this command to arouse all kinds of covetous desires within me! If there were no law, sin would not have that power. At one time I lived without understanding the law. But when I learned the command not to covet, for instance, the power of sin came to life, and I died. So

I discovered that the law's commands, which were supposed to bring life, brought spiritual death instead. Sin took advantage of those commands and deceived me; it used the commands to kill me. But still, the law itself is holy, and its commands are holy and right and good. But how can that be? Did the law, which is good, cause my death? Of course not! Sin used what was good to bring about my condemnation to death. So we can see how terrible sin really is. It uses God's good commands for its own evil purposes (Romans 7:4-13, NLT).

A few months after returning from this retreat, I spent my 23rd birthday at a strip club, which would very soon become my second home. Also around this time, my best friend, who had gone to Swaziland with me the previous summer, completely cut me off. I didn't understand why and I kept trying to figure out what I did wrong. My heart was completely devastated. Our friendship was one that grew from an awkward "don't touch me, don't make eye contact" to one that would cross many boundaries. Truly, I loved her more than anyone in the world at this time. We had become friends my sophomore year, her junior year of college, and she soon became my best and only friend. When we were together, nothing and no one else mattered, so I pushed many people away.

Her presence was hypnotizing. I felt completely safe when I was with her. No one could get to me, as long as I had her, I didn't need any other friends. I also knew I never wanted to be on the other side of this friendship. There was something about her I never quite could put my finger on, and this intrigued me. Capable of turning off emotions just as easily as flipping a switch, she cut me off. And I never felt a deeper pain or resentment from anyone, ever. I knew how cold she was capable of being, and I never expected to be on the receiving end of this. I couldn't fix it. I couldn't get past the wall she put up. I never knew it was possible for someone to completely change their demeanor, to go from loving and being protective, even jealous over you, to being able to look at you and act as if you never existed.

This Sadness- Tumblr, November 2013
I have never felt like this before. I can't shake it. It is bor-dering depression it is an immense sadness a bitter cold that seeps so deeply into my bones yet is never cold enough to freeze these tears that so easily fall. Anything can trigger them these days. And that is how I know I am still okay. When the tears no longer fall, I will then have to question whether there is anything left to fight for at all.

I was completely oblivious to many things during my college years, such as the strange texts in the middle of the night that I knew were not "her" writing, or the convulsing in my room while my family had a worship night one night in Swaziland, or the eyes. In the beginning of our friendship I wasn't allowed to look into her eyes for too long before she would look away. She started to teach me how to read eyes. I tried in the beginning and became frustrated though she said I had what it takes. I started to get it, but something didn't feel right- I got scared and decided I would leave eye-reading to her. Though I was scared of her, I saw brokenness underneath all of this that I so desperately wanted to fix. I wanted to be the friend she never had, to help heal all of the places that were hurt or broken.

I don't think I managed to do any of the above; surely, I am not God. But I had become so dependent on her, I wasn't even sure how to go on without her in my life. I walked around school like a lost puppy for months, trying at all costs to avoid her, while everything in me just wanted her to love me again. I suppose I wanted to be her god, and she had become mine in a way. I still do not understand many things about this friendship, but I do know that God was involved. I do know that He kept me, protected me from a lot. While my head was in the clouds and my heart blindly frolicking, brushing things off, rationalizing events that I didn't quite understand, there was a spiritual war going on and even in my oblivion, His hand was upon my life. He held me in my brokenness as I brokenly tried to hold another one of His dearly loved and broken sheep.

This past year there have been a few times I thought I saw her, and my heart nearly beat entirely out of my chest. I was deathly afraid of running into her for months. I have decided that if I ever were to run into her, I want to apologize. I wasn't a very good friend. And I was too lost to love in the right way. Too lost to realize that in my broken state, I could never help. I wasn't there when I needed to be. I was prideful, selfish, and completely blind to the fact that no one in this earth is capable of repairing another person's broken spirit, no matter how strong or good your intentions. We are all broken and in desperate need of a Savior. He loves her just as much as He loves me. He will win her heart.

Even When It Hurts- 2013
even when the sun's warmth sends shivers down your spine
and the clouds provide no comfort
no shelter for you to hide
even when a hug feels distant
and distant feels near
when the memories hurt so bad
and you wonder how you got here

when your current and constant heartache
is from a past you cannot erase or piece back together
when you worry how long this is taking
because you know there is no such thing as forever
when you fear tomorrow will come
because it only means one more day to dwell on yesterday
when you drink so much
yet cannot seem to drink the pain away
when you cry so hard you can barely open your eyes
when you no longer love to live
but you live to survive
when your heart becomes so heavy
and you feel you can no longer carry this burden
take one more step, you are not alone
together we are living and we are learning

CHAPTER 11: #WHITEGIRLDREADS

I was scrolling through Facebook one day, while waiting for my clothes to dry, and came across the FB page of someone who had graduated a few years before I even started at Notre Dame. I had heard about her before- she played basketball, could rap, and had been quite popular (or unpopular depending on who you asked) with the ladies. My heart was still hurting from my best friend cutting me off and I was struggling with making other friends as the closer I had become to her, the more I isolated myself from everyone else. When I came across her page, I saw posts about Jesus and about all He was doing in her life, and my heart jumped with excitement. I had to message her and find out more.

23/02/2014 23:13 Me
Whenever you have time...can I possibly talk to you about something? I know you don't really know me...but I think we may have a lot in common...and it would really be helpful to have someone to talk to right now who understands what I'm going through. Have a lovely night! God bless!

24/02/2014 12:16 Her
Yeah that sounds cool. I'm always up for good conversation.
26/02/2014 05:03 Her

Good morning. I hope you're having a good day. Just wanted to let you know you're in my prayers

26/02/2014 10:23 Me
Thank you so much.
Sorry I haven't hit you up yet this week has been a little rough...
Can I ask you something?

26/02/2014 11:00 Her
It's all good. Sure go ahead

26/02/2014 11:06 Me
Okay... not really sure how to ask this lol. Are you/were you a lesbian?

26/02/2014 14:10 Her
Lol. Yes I was a lesbian. I dated girls for about 5 years. Then when I accepted Jesus as my Lord and Savior I felt really convicted about being with girls. Honestly it's still something I struggle with in a lot of ways

26/02/2014 14:15 Me
Sorry if that was weird. Okay, well I'm going through the same thing, well similar, so I figured I'd ask you about it. I was brought up in a Christian family...my whole life in church...my parents are actually missionaries in southern Africa, but when I was like 13 I started crushing on my friends and when I was 17 came out and broke my family's heart. I got kicked out of leadership at church... was in a lot of ways hurt by the church and because of some of the treatment I got I pushed God completely out of my life, though I always felt Him trying to pull me back. Since I was little I felt a call on my life...I don't know what His plan is but I know it is big and when I pushed Him away 6 years ago I felt I lost that...and I looked to girls, over and over again to fill that void in my life that only He could fill. And every relationship or sexual encounter left me feel-

ing...well gratified in a way...for a short period of time...but always the same result: more emptiness and less of my heart left. I think it all started when I had a few friends I knew were lesbians and I tried to "save them" or be God to them and from there I slipped in...and tried to "fix" the brokenness in girls and when I myself was broken I went to girls I saw as stronger than myself for them to "fix me", but this past year I have felt God so strongly to the point where I could no longer deny He was real no matter how hard I tried, and I did try lol. He never gave up trying to get through to me...and it took me reaching my breaking point to realize that, but now I feel, I don't know....scared.

26/02/2014 14:20 Her
Lol no worries. I can definitely relate to so much of what you're saying it's scary

26/02/2014 14:20 Me
I'm terrified. Like I have spent the past 5 years or so creating this identity...and I know I need to find my identity in Him alone, but I feel so scared.

26/02/2014 14:21 Her
And now you feel like you have to rebuild who you are?

26/02/2014 14:21 Me
Yes...and I don't know where to start. I have been praying for someone or a mentor or something because I feel there aren't too many people who can really understand...I found a church that I really like and the women there are amazing and have been praying with and for me but I don't know. It would be so much easier just to stay this way, just to give in to the desires of my flesh, but I know that would mean giving up everything God has in store...and I don't want that. I want to live with purpose and for Him to fulfill the desires of my heart in His way and timing. Sometimes I wish I would have had any other kind of struggle besides this one...it's not easy

when it has become so deeply intertwined with who you are.

26/02/2014 14:25 Her
I have found myself saying the same thing. And in a society where it is made out to be normal.

26/02/2014 14:25 Me
Yes. And I don't know if I could ever be okay with telling my gay friends that this is wrong when I have defended it and fought for it for so long.

26/02/2014 14:25 Her
Yeah, but I think what God is doing in your life is beautiful. And it really fills my heart with joy to hear that you want to follow Jesus.

The first few times we hung out were very encouraging. We shared our testimonies and shared what God was teaching us in His word. However, rather than holding each other accountable and getting plugged into fellowship outside of ourselves, we were focusing too much on a list of do's and don'ts and were completely missing the point of grace. We were still both struggling individually, and would soon be in all of the places we were trying to leave behind, together. I would drag her into strip clubs, later to find out that the times she would seem to randomly disappear, she was actually in the bathroom crying because though we were usually drunk and having fun, she knew even in this state that she was not supposed to be in there.

It wasn't that I didn't know, I just pretended to ignore it. The more conviction I felt, the more I drank, the more I needed to be distracted. I had gotten dreadlocks a year before we met, partially because I had always wanted them and partially because my best friend at that time had locs and I wanted everyone to know I was with her. I soon found out that they seemed to be an asset in getting attention from other women.

She got locs, too, and in all of our IG pictures we proudly presented ourselves as #whitegirldreads. We would go out to the gay clubs and parties together, and were always looking for new ladies to talk to, the more attention we had, the better we felt about ourselves. I comforted her when her heart was broken and she did the same for me. She very quickly became like a sister and best friend to me, and I praise God that even while we were blindly leading each other down a very destructive path, His hand was still evident in our lives. I praise God for the times she would sit me down and ask how much longer we were going to do this, the times she tried to take a stand, though I wasn't ready to hear it. He spoke to me through her words so many times. Seeds were planted. We had to go through the fire together, I suppose, in order to be able to be there to support and hold each other accountable in coming out.

Beautifully Broken- August 2014
Sometimes my eyes give all away
And sometimes they tell absolutely nothing at all
Sometimes I feel so strongly through them
I can't help but shut them and let a few tears fall

I am no good at voicing my feelings
I'd rather put them all down in words
Let these hands write type strum them
till they are tired till the fear subsides
or till my every fingertip hurts

If only I was not so very human

If only pain was a little less real
I would strum away forever
I'd write till I ran out of paper
till I ran out of words or till I had nothing left to feel

If ever you think you cannot read me
If ever I seem distracted aloof or far
It is only because I am fighting off my demons
Fear being the worst one
The one that kills me
The one that makes expressing myself so hard

It seems such a simple concept opening your mouth letting words flow
out
But I want every word to be of substance
So I calculate profusely
As the moment passes
And I am overcome with doubt

I'm trying to trust Him because I've grown weary and am still learn-
ing to trust my own heart
But this is hard when it has so often failed me and I have not yet fully
mastered my guard

I long to be broken open in a way that is beautiful
For this unsteady wall to come crumbling down
For wisdom and His heart to guide me so that I am not always afraid
I will fall

And when I do fall it will be for good reason and I will find my voice
again

I trust the disconnect between heart and mouth can be mended

I trust that He works all things out for good in the end

CHAPTER 12: IT HAS ALL BECOME TOO MUCH

I am not quite sure how I passed nursing school, to be perfectly honest. I have always done well in school, and I did put a lot of time into studying and completing my work, but I truly am not sure when I found time to do my work and study in between and in the midst of everything else. I gave up soccer during my junior year, because nursing school had become too intense and when I did have extra time I was speedily getting my work done so that I could spend the evenings and weekend partying and at the club. As most places usually shut down around 2, I became a regular at the afterhours spot, 1722, which allowed us to continue the party until about 5am.

I began spending most weekends at my older friends' house and was introduced to polyamory, the swinger scene, and various drugs, which I usually had no trouble denying. One night in particular, I met up with the crew, and we went to a swinger's club. While in the bathroom, I kissed one of them. I'm pretty sure I knew she had LSD in her mouth, which was then transferred to mine. LSD combined with whiskey and all I remember from the club was how colorful everything was. How out of control everything felt. How that night when we were finally back at their house, no matter how I tried, I could not relax, I could not for the life of me go to sleep, though I was exhausted.

The next morning, my friends, who I do not believe ever meant to harm me in any way, decided to have a little fun with me. I was the youngest in our group, and I wanted them to think I was just as tough, just as daring, just as sexy, so though I could have very well said no, to many things, I usually just convinced myself this was what living was about. Taking risks. Even when it hurt. YOLO. Their approval was worth it. That day, I allowed something to happen that I thought only hurt physically, but had long term emotional ramifications as well. I never told them this of course, I just slowly distanced myself. It wasn't their fault that I couldn't stand for anything, particularly myself.

During my last few years of college, when I was there, I was distracted. When I was not there, I was on a date, trying to be on a date, or somewhere drinking. I became a regular at one of the strip clubs in downtown Baltimore and began talking to one of the dancers there. I started spending a lot of time with her, often skipping multiple days of school at a time. I made it my priority to be at the club anytime she was working, which was most nights. I would go to watch her dance and also to make sure no one else was watching too long. The jealousy I felt when they did was infuriating.

She had to constantly remind me that this was her job, though this was not very comforting, because I realized I couldn't distinguish between show and reality. I would wait for her to get off of work around 3am, promising myself, every time that I was not going to drink, as I sometimes had to be at clinical the next morning at 6:30am. I wasn't the best at keeping promises, and I needed something to distract me from my jealous rage and insecurity. I began smoking even more and drinking heavily. At this point I had also begun working part time night shift at a hospital as a tech, so I truly do not understand how I managed to work, sleep, do my school work, and survive clinicals in between being with her or at the club.

I wanted to be wherever she was. I would beg her not to go to work some nights so I could take her on dates. Walking around with her on my arm, I felt invincible. I felt special. I knew she was struggling and had dreams of being somewhere else, doing something else, but she didn't like to stay sober long enough to pursue any of that. While drunk one night, she slipped and told me she loved me. Strangely, for me, I could not say it back. I did love her. But somewhere deep inside I knew this was not going to last very long and I knew I could not let any more of my heart go than I had already given. Being with her, while it definitely was a constant adrenaline rush, was beginning to feel more and more dangerous. I felt like we were always hiding. She was always hiding me, not so much worried about herself but what someone might do to me. I knew she had been in a relationship before we met, but I didn't know the extent of it.

There came a point where she let me know she was actually in a relationship the whole time and her girlfriend, or wife, whichever she was, found out she was talking to me. She waited for her to get off work one night and beat her up pretty bad. I was at work when she called me, screaming and crying, as her girlfriend stood outside the house trying to beat down the door. I nearly left work I was so worried about her, but she made me promise to stay. The next day I tried to reach her all day but her phone was off. I drove halfway to her house and turned around 2 or 3 times.

Finally, she answered the phone and I was able to talk her into riding with me to a dentist appointment. She agreed to go if I would pick her up a few streets over from her house just to be safe, in case her girlfriend was watching. My heart hurt watching her limp to my car, but when she opened the door and slowly inched her way into the seat, wincing in pain, and I saw the cuts, the bruises up her arms, around her neck, her swollen eyes and lips…my heart couldn't bear it. I had to turn away for a good minute or two and get myself together.

After this, she made me stay away for a while, but, not able to take a hint, I eventually returned, pretended nothing had changed. All the while, the questions tormented me. I couldn't understand how someone who claimed to love her could treat her the way she did, or how someone who claimed to love me could lie and be in a relationship the entire time, even now after being treated that way. These thoughts didn't plague me so long as I was drunk.

When I looked at her, though I was broken myself, I saw someone I knew was hurting and had been hurt far deeper than I ever had. Someone who wanted things to be different so that her 14 year old daughter might be able to have a chance at life like she never had, but she couldn't seem to break the cycle. And I longed with everything inside me to be able to heal that brokenness, to be able to offer hope. Yet I knew I didn't have what it took. And I knew when she looked at me, underneath the drunkenness and the show, she couldn't bear the thought of seeing me become trapped in this cycle of pain with her.

I somewhat realized that it was probably not in anyone's best interest for us to continue talking after I awoke abruptly one morning to the sound of her girlfriend banging on the doors and windows threatening to kill whoever was in the house with her. She pushed me into a closet full of empty vodka and whiskey bottles, as I stood there hung-over, wondering what was surrounding me in this closet, and afraid for my life.

Later that day when she called and told me she loved me but she loved her girlfriend and wanted to try to make it work, I was furious. I shouted at her and cursed her as I cried angry, broken tears, not understanding but knowing deep inside that this was always how it was going to end. That it had to end. We stopped talking, and I spent the next few months drinking and occasionally somehow ending up back at the strip club, only to always leave in tears. Despite all of the issues and drama, most of which I cannot even discuss here, for some reason, she had a hold on me I found extremely difficult and painful to shake.

It Has All Become Too Much- July 2014
Pulling away from it all, because it has all become too much.
I fear my longing to fall in love has become both my weakness and my crutch.
I hurt when I am hurting I don't mean to cut you with my tongue.
I am not one to inflict pain on even those who break me I think something inside has been left unsung
for far too long this has been slowly building and with each new hurt I continue to find,
I am not really going much of anywhere but I am constantly losing my mind.
Still not sure of who I am but always worried of who I'm becoming
I wonder if it would do me better to stop where I've fallen or to close my eyes and just keep running.
Towards what, I am uncertain, I feel my passion is beginning to

fade
perhaps that's just my sundered soul rambling or perhaps I have
finally fallen in the bed I have made.
I know I have so much yet to live for a purpose much greater
than my own
but it is so easy to get distracted when my heart is constantly
longing to find a home.
I am not ready to love or be loved, I know this, and I have finally realized,
that not every person who shows you attention is worth your
downfall,
worth that last sparkle in your eyes.
I want to be the best me I can be
not this fragile butterfly,
who is so lost I refuse to tell the difference
between wisdom and blatant lies.
I am not this broken individual I have lately portrayed myself to
be,
through my stupidity and poor judgment, my inability to see
what everyone else sees.
So I am pulling away from it all because I have made it all too
much.
I am going to work on loving myself, walk this path on my own,
without a crutch.

CHAPTER 13: WHAT WAS MEANT FOR EVIL

A few months after this relationship, after many poems, cry sessions, and speeches about how I'm not dating anyone ever again because I need to get to know myself, I began talking to someone else. I had actually met her a year before this, at a lesbian club in D.C. where I was standing at the bar alone and visibly upset because my girlfriend at the time had hurt my feelings. She approached me and asked if I was okay, which of course made my girlfriend all of the sudden care. That conversation didn't last too long, but I never forgot about her kindness in checking on me that random night at the bar. We were dating after a few weeks of talking and I was very soon spending every weekend in Washington, D.C.

She was also raised in a Christian home, and her sister, like mine, just happened to be an on-fire, and anointed woman of God, in Bible School in Louisiana. We went out most weekends, to different lesbian clubs around D.C., and also were members of a church, that predominantly catered to the LGBT community. I met some of the most loving people at this church, who will always hold a special place in my heart and in my prayers. For the first time in a very long time, I began to seek God again. I began journaling from time to time, but our lifestyle, apart from church on Sunday mornings, was not in any way, shape, or form reflecting the God we were seeking. Our sisters, who have been and still are our prayer warriors continued to speak truth into our lives, though it only made us angry and hurt. We still were not ready to listen.

Let Me- October 2014
Life is so much bigger than you think you know what love means
What it feels how it touches the heart of another and the implications
of this gentle reminder that
You have not a clue.
Yet you let it consume you
are lost
In love
In lust
In your own human desires that have never been about
Me.
I want to use you mold you make you Holy show you how
Love loves
But you
Get so caught up
In things that at the end of this journey will amount to nothing
And here I am
Have been
Will be
Standing
Arms open
Offering so much more than you ever gave Me time to show you...
This gift is surrender.
This path requires ultimate sacrifice.
You will be lonely
But you are Never alone
I have Never let you go

Do not Ever
Believe that lie
I am Always by your side
I have Beautiful plans for your Whole life.
And if tomorrow is the day you die...
...if you just let Me
Let you
Fall
I have hold
Trust that I alone Am
in complete Control...
You need not fear nor fret
For My Love means Eternal Salvation for your Soul.

Journal- January 2015
He tugs and I run away further and further every time I get lost in the daily the rush in the struggle I wrestle my own heart to the ground and forget how much more sense life makes with Him involved. It's easy to forget sometimes though I can hardly blame the absence of mind my mind knows full well what it does yet I'll continue to blame...because...well, that just works for me. As do many things as of late. Many things I know in my heart of hearts need fixing repaired made new reversed erased. Cleanse my mind soften my heart help to remember what and Who is true. Because there has never been a day moment or second that I, in all of my extravagant failure, have ever escaped You.

About 9 months into our relationship, she went to Louisiana, to a conference at her sister's church. A week prior to this she told me she had a dream where her mom, who had passed away a few years earlier, had told her that we were not going to be in each other's lives the way we thought. When she told me this, my heart sank. It felt as if the numbness I had built up the past few years had begun to melt and that conviction was setting back in. During this conference, she experienced God in a very special way and while she was away I sensed this.

I sensed that things were about to be shaken up, so I did what I knew would help dissipate the fear in my heart. I went back to the strip club. I drank. I tried not to think about what was coming. When she returned she let me know she had taken a purity vow. I was slightly shocked, but I respected this, of course. It was after this was no longer a factor in our relationship that God began to truly speak to both of our hearts. It did not feel like love and butterflies. It felt like I was preparing for death. We didn't understand what was coming yet. But God had made it clear to her while she was in LA that she was supposed to be in New Orleans, in Bible school.

About a month after this, in March of 2015, it was about that time for my 24th birthday. We went to a restaurant and casino and I drank way too much. I distinctly remember feeling such heaviness in my heart that whole night. I woke up the next morning and for all intents and purposes- minus the hangover, I should have been "happy." I had a great birthday, celebrating with all of my friends, and my girlfriend was next to me. It was a beautiful Sunday morning.

However, my heart felt so heavy I could do nothing but cry. She, confused, began to try to figure out what was wrong. The only thing I could get out, through painful, heart wrenching sobs was, "I don't know if we can be gay and Christian and you're leaving me". I'm pretty sure she laughed at me in my pitiful, snotty state, and tried to reassure me that I was overthinking things, as usual. She was not as upset as I was, because at this point I don't think she understood what was about to happen- thinking perhaps we could hold on, to both our relationship and the call of God on our lives. We watched a sermon online that morning, which only further confirmed what God was speaking to my heart.

After the sermon was over, she went to shower, and I called my mom on Skype. As soon as she answered, the floodgates broke open and I sat there and wept. My mom cried with me, though for a while I was not even able to utter a coherent word through my sobs. Finally, I managed to catch my breath and I was somewhat able to explain what I was crying about. I think she already knew. My mom prayed with me and though crying, seemed to be relieved that I was finally coming to this realization, but I could feel her heart breaking with mine. Come to find out, 9 months earlier, my mom was devastated when she found out I was in yet another relationship. However, it was in this place God met her and made it very clear to her that He was going to use this relationship to not only bring me back to Him, but to bring us both back to Him. I think our moms were in on this together.

CHAPTER 14: THE RETURN

"My heart has heard you say, "Come and talk with me." And
my heart responds, "LORD, I am coming.""
Psalms 27:8

The next few weeks were some of the most painful weeks of my life thus far. At first I tried to fight, again. This time, I got sick. For two weeks I was so sick I could barely get out of bed to go to the bathroom, much less feed myself. My grandparents had to come pick me up from campus and take care of me at home, just to make sure I was eating. At one point I called my sister, terrified, and gasping for breath, to ask her to pray with me because my throat was so swollen I could barely breathe. It was in these two weeks that God really ministered to my heart. I had no choice. I couldn't get out of bed. I couldn't drink. I couldn't run to the club. I couldn't hop on the train to D.C., and my girlfriend's car was having issues so she couldn't come see me. I just had to lay there. And think. And listen.

I finally had the strength to return to my dorm, and the night I did, there was an event being put on by Bethel Campus Fellowship (BCF), called Gethsemane Experience. I had seen signs around campus talking about it, but I wasn't planning on going. I was still running fever, and I was an hour late, but as I lay there, God very clearly told me to get up and go. So I went. When I walked in, they were finishing up the sermon and the verse on the screen was: Then Jesus said, "Come to me, all of you who are weary and carry heavy burdens, and I will give you rest" (Matthew 11:28). I instantly began crying. When the sermon was over they said that all of those who need prayer can stay behind. I stayed.

Two of the BCF leaders talked and prayed with me. They reminded me that God does not cause confusion and the fact that I was confused about being gay clearly meant there was no peace. No one had said anything that night about being gay. So where was it coming from? One told me she sensed the burdens I was carrying as soon as I walked in, and that God wanted me to surrender them. I gave my life back to Christ that night, and I knew this time was going to be different. I meant every word of my prayer with every ounce of my heart that was left. Exhausted from running, worn from the pain and hurt of the past 8 years, I gave up fighting the One who only ever offered me love. When I asked Him to forgive me, I meant it. When I asked Him to help, I needed it. I knew it would not be sunshine and daisies moving forward.

One of the women who prayed with me would become a mentor. Over the next few weeks she would text, call, meet me for lunch and Bible study, constantly asking "how is your heart", "what is He saying to you?" There would be days that I would feel like giving up and running straight back to my comfort zone, so I would avoid her calls, avoid bumping into her. However, when she started showing up to my dorm room, I knew getting away from God wasn't going to be an easy feat this time around. I thank God for her life every day. Knowing He loved me enough to send someone into my life to make sure I knew I wasn't forgotten, to make sure I knew I had someone to reach out to, to walk through this with me, it kept me going. It strengthened my heart.

Those few weeks were incredibly hard because it had become very clear to me that in order for my girlfriend to make the decision to go to Bible School, in order for us both to be able to heal, to come back to Christ, I needed to make a complete cut. This was painful, because I loved her still, and she did not understand why I was doing it. I stayed with my best friend for a few weeks, because I knew if I stayed alone in my dorm room I would give in and just go to D.C. to make her feel better.

My best friend was also walking away from homosexuality at this time, so we spent many nights crying, but trying to encourage each other. The urgency we felt this time around was so very strong. As mentioned earlier, she had occasionally brought up over the past year how she felt God was calling us out of this lifestyle, but I was always quick to change the subject or argue that we could very simply combine both lives. When God got a hold of me and I was the one saying it's time, she knew this was serious.

I had to make a decision and stick with it, and pray God would work on my girlfriend's heart just as He was working on mine. And He did. I had to remember that He was pursuing her heart just as much as He was pursuing mine. He was taking care of her, too. If you are struggling to let go of someone, please remember that He loves them so much more than you ever could. That is a tough thing to remember when all you can feel is the pain of letting go, when you are sure that person cannot survive without you. They can. And they will. He will meet them in their place of brokenness just as He is meeting you in yours.

During this time there were a few verses I meditated on daily, because when you lay down or walk away from something, without replacing that void with Him, as I had done a few years prior, it is way too easy to fall. We are at war, spiritually, and our minds are so easily distracted and swayed if we are not grounded in Jesus. Thoughts raced through my mind constantly. I was terrified of being alone, both in the sense that I did not like to be alone with my thoughts and in the sense that I did not even know what it was to be on my own, completely emotionally and spiritually unattached to another human being. I was scared of what I would find the longer I spent time with myself. I was scared of failing. I was scared of what people would think or say, of being called closed-minded, fake, or hateful. You name it, and I was scared of it. I was very much so aware of the power of the mind, but I had yet to learn the power of His love, in casting out fear:

There is no fear in love. But perfect love drives out fear, because fear has to do with punishment. The one who fears is not made perfect in love (1 John 4:18, NLT).

But now, O Jacob, listen to the LORD who created you. O Israel, the one who formed you says, "Do not be afraid, for I have ransomed you. I have called you by name; you are mine. When you go through deep waters, I will be with you. When you go through rivers of difficulty, you will not drown. When you walk through the fire of oppression, you will not be burned up; the flames will not consume you. For I am the LORD, your God, the Holy One of Israel, your Savior. I gave Egypt as a ransom for your freedom; I gave Ethiopia and Seba in your place. Others were given in exchange for you. I traded their lives for yours because you are precious to me. You are honored, and I love you.

Do not be afraid, for I am with you. I will gather you and your children from east and west (Isaiah 43:1-5, NLT).

And then, in giving us the strength to hold these thoughts captive so that they do not control us:

For though we live in the world, we do not wage war as the world does. The weapons we fight with are not the weapons of the world. On the contrary, they have divine power to demolish strongholds. We demolish arguments and every pretension that sets itself up against the knowledge of God, and we take captive every thought to make it obedient to Christ (2 Corinthians 10:3-5, NIV).

Don't worry about anything; instead, pray about everything. Tell God what you need, and thank him for all he has done. Then you will experience God's peace, which exceeds anything we can understand. His peace will guard your hearts and minds as you live in Christ Jesus. And now, dear brothers and sisters, one final thing. Fix your thoughts on what is true, and honorable, and right, and pure, and lovely, and admirable. Think about things that are excellent and worthy of praise. Keep putting into practice all you learned and received from me—everything you heard from me and saw me doing. Then the God of peace will be with you (Philippians 4:6-9, NLT).

Journal- May 2015
Even when I break Your heart
You're always near You're never far
Though time may pass and distance grow
My mind still wavers to and fro
I linger on things and people and times

When I was not living for You
But for my own selfish high
The attention I sought, Your gentle voice I angrily fought
Blaming You for this pain, when it was completely my fault.
You did nothing but love me.
You do nothing but love me.
You are here now, You love me.
Though I doubt, You still love me.
With or without, You will love me.
And when the whole world ceases to be
When breathing stops and I can finally see
You face to face
I will drop to my knees
For I was never worthy
But You still loved me.

After being invited numerous times, my best friend and I finally decided to visit a church called CAC Bethel Baltimore. The Saturday night before going to church, we both tossed and turned and tried to think of any and every excuse possible as to why we couldn't go to church. Driving there, we almost turned around twice, stopped for coffee, and then ended up going to the wrong church. The people there were very friendly, but when we told them who invited us and they responded by asking who that was, we knew something was off. We thanked them for their hospitality, promised to visit one day, and continued this very eventful journey to church, posting an instagram picture displaying are terrified faces before finally making our way inside.

I do not consider myself yet to have taken hold of it. But one thing I do: Forgetting what is behind and straining toward what

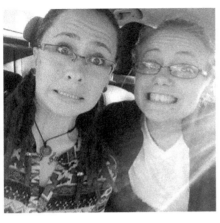

is ahead (Philippians 3:13, NIV).

I do not even remember what the service was about that day. My heart was so overwhelmed and my mind was going 100 miles a minute trying to take everything in. After the service, we were invited into one of the meeting rooms and the young adult group surrounded us as we shared a little bit of what was going on in our lives, what God was doing. Each and every person came up to us and hugged us and told us we were loved. They shared their stories with us, their struggles, and how God has delivered.

Our hearts were so overwhelmed with love. We didn't feel alone anymore. We were part of a family of others who also struggled and struggle, but have learned to cling to Jesus with all they have. I love how God works. I had been whining about being homesick, and while Nigeria is not Swaziland, I still find it funny that I am now members of a church of Nigerian origin. He takes care of the big and the little things in our lives. He cares about all of it. I am in awe, constantly. We went to breakfast after church and sat there dumbfounded at what had just happened. It was all I could do not to burst into tears, my heart was so full.

Rest- June 2015
At peace knowing He understands me better than I do myself. Knowing that He sees me, He knows me, and He cares. About even the parts of my life I deem insignificant and unwor-

thy of attention.

If there is one thing He has taught me over the past few weeks, it is this: Though I am stubborn. Though I am needy. Though I like to maintain control even if it's just a string to hold onto...

He allows me wiggle room but never so much as to cut me loose and I appreciate that so very much. Because it is this perfect Love that leaves me completely speechless and in awe at the end of each and every day when I realize that His plan is always higher. Always greater. Always better than anything I thought I had control of or tried to make happen in my own strength and limited insight.

His Love is what I live for. His Love gives me butterflies, goosebumps, and takes my breath away. His love brings me to my knees. And in this Love...

I will rest.

CHAPTER 15: FIGHT

God has done so much in my life in the past year. Too much to even do justice in writing. However, it has not been easy. There have been many days where I have felt like throwing in the towel. I made a promise to God when I first came back to Him that I would never mess up again. I very quickly realized that this was an incredibly dumb promise to make. Thankfully, He does not think the way we do. Thankfully, He knew before I did that it was a dumb promise.

A few months into walking with Christ, with a new job and the start of grad school, I became too busy for God. I became too comfortable with my daily routine, and it got to the point where He was no longer a part of it. Therefore, my peace was quickly fading and all of these worries and doubts started to make their way back into my heart. Before you know it, I was feeling lonely and out of control and I wanted to be in control again. So I did what I knew had in the past made me feel in control. I made an OKCupid account- a 'Christian version', and looking at men this time instead of women. I somehow convinced myself this was okay, but soon realized that the fact that I was scared to tell my best friend and mentors about it probably meant that I knew deep down that this was me trying to do God's job, yet again.

I met a guy, who said he was a Christian and had been involved in ministry in Kenya. He must be the one! He asked me to lunch one day after church and I said yes, though I really didn't feel peace about going. It was an interesting date- we went for a run and then to lunch and ice cream. On my way home, I had a slight melt down. He was a great guy, very sweet, loves the Lord, but I wasn't attracted to him. Rather than let this confirm the obvious- which was that he simply was not the one- I decided that it meant I was doomed to be single my whole life. That I was not, nor would I ever, be attracted to men. And therefore, I clearly had to go back to what I knew.

The next day I responded to a message from someone I had been interested in about a year prior, who I had also met on OKCupid. At the time we had been talking, we were trying to plan her coming to Baltimore to visit for a weekend. A year later, we proceeded to schedule this visit and I did my best to keep myself busy all week, avoiding my mentors and best friend, because I could already feel God tugging on my heart without the addition of their words of wisdom.

Before I knew it, it was Friday evening and she texted me to let me know she was in my driveway. My heart sank. My prayer in this moment: "God, I know I messed up. I know I'm messing up. Please, please don't let me fall harder than I am able to recover from". And with that we commenced a weekend filled with wine, movies I did not need to be watching, bars, and art museums. There were times she would ask me about my faith or what God had done in my life over the past few months, because she had seen my Facebook. She knew I had walked away from this life, yet here I was, guzzling wine in attempts to block His voice and correction, as I returned to being the flirt I had been just months before. When she asked, I avoided the topic.

I felt like Peter must have felt when people asked him about His association with Jesus, and he wholeheartedly denied it. Then, Jesus looked at him and his heart was crushed. I knew I was breaking His heart, as well as confusing another one of His sheep. So much more could have happened this weekend than did happen- I am not sure if it was Him protecting me, or merely the fact that it had become harder for me to fully return to my old ways, perhaps a combination of the two. On Sunday morning she decided she needed to leave early, which left me sitting alone in my room, with time to reflect. With nothing to show for the weekend except a headache, I buried my face in my pillow and cried. I was angry. I was ashamed. And I couldn't bring myself to speak to the One who only wanted me, even after all of my disobedience, to simply cry out to Him.

It was 8am. Church started at 9. I wasn't going.

I texted my mentors, my best friend, and my mom and told them all I was never going to church again, I was a failure, I was giving up, and I was going to hide in a cave, so they should all forget about me (because that's exactly what one does when they decide they want to disappear). Of course, they ALL called me and told me to get my butt to church. I pitifully put on the outfit I had worn the night before, not particularly caring that it was one of the outfits I used to wear when I was trying to appear more masculine. I cried the whole way there, and then sat in the parking lot on the curb for 30 minutes, because I did not want to go inside and tell anyone what had just happened. Two of my friends just happened to be late that day and found me sobbing on the curb next to my car. They immediately joined me, wrapped their arms around me, and began praying for me. My mentor came outside and joined us and rather than lecture me or drill me on what had just happened, he just hugged me and prayed.

There was a guest minister that morning and when they walked me in, the song she was singing surrounded me and I felt the presence of God so strongly.

I want to fall in love with You all over again. Help me to fall in love with You. Sweet Jesus, sweet Savior, Creator of everything.

I fell to my knees, tears and snot everywhere, and cried out to Jesus to hold me, to heal me, to forgive me. I knew I had messed up, but more than anything I knew I had broken His heart, and consciously, on purpose. Yet, I didn't feel condemned by Him. The more I cried out to Him, the more I felt His love rush over me, and the burden begin to lift. The lady who was ministering, along with my mentors, took me, in all of my crying glory, to the back room for prayer. She looked at me, took my face in her hands, and rather than see her when I looked up, I truly felt like God was looking into my heart through her. She allowed God to use her to speak some words into my situation, truth that I will never, ever forget.

It completely blows my mind that even when I went out of my way to completely disobey and deny Him, He would send someone not to convey a message of condemnation or anger, but simply to remind me that to Him, I am beautiful. That He didn't make a mistake when He made me, beautifully feminine, and more than enough. That He loves me. That I am accepted by Him. And that He is healing the pain of every rejection I had ever experienced.

Journal- September 2015
My heart is not capable of the depth of love You deserve. I

break Your heart on purpose still You run to pick me up. I cannot fathom Your love, Your mercy, Your forgiveness...I cannot fathom You. But I thank You.

You see, homosexuality was not something I was delivered from in the sense that I woke up one morning and all feelings, desires, thoughts were completely gone. Not at all. Like any struggle or sin, it is a daily death to self and surrender to Him. This just happens to be my weakness. And if it is my weakness every day for the rest of my life, that is okay, because it keeps me close to Him. I love the verse where Paul talks about the thorn in his side:

Three different times I begged the Lord to take it away. Each time he said, "My grace is all you need. My power works best in weakness." So now I am glad to boast about my weaknesses, so that the power of Christ can work through me. That's why I take pleasure in my weaknesses, and in the insults, hardships, persecutions, and troubles that I suffer for Christ. For when I am weak, then I am strong (2 Corinthians 12:8-10, NLT).

I am constantly reminded how tightly I have to cling to Him. And that is exactly where I want and need to be. In full dependence. It is truly humbling realizing that it is in our greatest weakness that He is able to impart greatest strength on us. As long as we keep close. It is easy to go back to what is "comfortable" in moments of weakness or fear, when we let the busyness and chaos of life take the place of Him and do not spend enough time in His presence. You can only go for so long without a refill before the flesh begins to creep its way back in. Through falling over the past few months, I learned a few very important lessons:

1.   Though He has done a great work in my life and I truly do feel like a new person, I am not immune to falling, which is why I have to stay close.

2.   Because my old life was full of all kinds of sin, there are certain things I simply cannot listen to, places I cannot go, people I cannot associate with, and things I cannot watch. This does not make me weak, well actually it does, but there is strength in realizing it, in asking for help, and in self-control.

3.   His grace is STILL sufficient.

4.   Even when I go out of my way to slap Him in the face, He goes out of His to show Love.

I love the word "redemption", mostly because of the "re", which means that He already had us. He created us- we have always, always been His. But because of sin, we were separated. He could not bear for us to be separate from Him. He longs for fellowship with us- this is why we were created. He didn't simply leave us in our mess. He bought us back. Again. With a ransom, a purchase, a rescue, to free us from the consequences of sin. The idea of my life being ransomed is something that makes my heart so overwhelmed with love. God, the Creator of Heaven and earth, loved me enough to pay a price for my life, the ultimate price, the life of His one and only Son, to demand my release from captivity. Simply so that I can fellowship with Him for all eternity. Simply because He loves me *that* much. Wow.

For God so loved the world that he gave his one and only Son, that whoever believes in him shall not perish but have eternal life. For God did not send his Son into the world to condemn the world, but to save the world through him (John 3:16-17, NIV).

John 3:16. Probably one of the most popular and well known verses. However, the part that I want to focus on is verse 17. That is the message of redemption. God sent His only Son into this world while we were still in sin, NOT to judge the world. Not to point fingers at us and tell all of our sins, secrets, issues, fears, and failures to the world. Not to remind us how much we fall short or mess up on a daily, no, minute-by-minute basis. Not to walk around in all of His glory and perfection, showing off or trying to make us feel bad for not being able to live up to God's standard of perfection. But to be the bridge, the final sacrifice, the lifeline that pulls us out of the brokenness and searching and emptiness we experience when we live a life apart from Him. When we have not yet truly experienced His heart for us.

But now God has shown us a way to be made right with him without keeping the requirements of the law, as was promised in the writings of Moses and the prophets long ago. We are made right with God by placing our faith in Jesus Christ. And this is true for everyone who believes, no matter who we are. For everyone has sinned; we all fall short of God's glorious standard. Yet God, with undeserved kindness, declares that we are righteous. He did this through Christ Jesus when he freed us from the penalty for our sins. For God presented Jesus as the sacrifice for sin. People are made right with God when they believe that Jesus sacrificed his life, shedding his blood. This sacrifice shows that God was being fair when he held back and did not punish those who sinned in times past, for he was looking ahead and including them in what he would do in this present time. God did this to demonstrate his righteousness, for he himself is fair and just, and he declares sinners to be right in his sight when they believe in Jesus (Romans 3:21-26, NLT).

God is not a forceful Lover. He is a gentleman, and He will never push Himself on you, regardless of how desperately you may need Him. He gives you the freedom to choose Love or to choose to do things your own way. When you choose Him, He will step in and fight with and for you. But it is a choice you have to make, and it will involve some rather painful action of letting go of things and people in order to make room for Him to take over. And even after you have chosen Him, there will be moments where you feel you have absolutely no strength left, no motivation to keep fighting, moments when it seems so much easier and less painful to go back.

You will have these moments, and when you do, stop. Pause every single one of those thoughts and doubts and fears, because they are not of God. They are the enemy trying his very hardest (which is nothing compared to the strength of your Savior) to make you feel worthless and weak. He wants to make you think you are fighting this alone, that you do not measure up, that you are not a child of God. Stop these thoughts before they go any further and pray this scripture over your mind:

For though we walk in the flesh, we do not war according to the flesh. For the weapons of our warfare are not carnal but mighty in God for pulling down strongholds, casting down arguments and every high thing that exalts itself against the knowledge of God, bringing every thought into captivity to the obedience of Christ, and being ready to punish all disobedience when your obedience is fulfilled (2 Corinthians 10:3-5, NKJV).

I cannot stress the importance of fellowship enough. Find a church and/or a small group where you can make friends, who are also walking with Christ and who you can be accountable to. A good friend of mine, whom I met at church, has been there for me at my lowest. When I am struggling I know I can message her and expect a text or a call within minutes, either to pray with or encourage me with scripture. One night, a few months into my walk, I texted her letting her know I was battling with thoughts of giving up. She sent me a prayer, which I prayed very often for the next few weeks:

Hey God, my past is looking better right now. I am afraid of the future and the challenges, but God I need Your perfect love to silence all of the lies in my head and I need a reassurance that You are with me. Lord, I know You are with me but I pray that You would show me You are near even in this moment. Father, I pray that You would forgive my unbelief. Amen.

It does not make you weak to ask for help. In fact, I consider vulnerability, as it is difficult and often uncomfortable, to be a great strength. It is crucial in this process, as you learn to walk with Christ. The Bible speaks on the importance of this in order for healing and restoration to take place:

Confess to one another therefore your faults (your slips, your false steps, your offenses, your sins) and pray [also] for one another, that you may be healed and restored [to a spiritual tone of mind and heart]. The earnest (heartfelt, continued) prayer of a righteous man makes tremendous power available [dynamic in its working] (James 5:16, AMP).

It is so important to remember that this journey is not measured by what you do or don't do. You cannot fight spiritual battles with physical warfare. It is only by the grace of God and because He is fighting for you that we overcome. He does not, nor has He ever expected you to fight this alone.

Plead my cause, O Lord, with those who strive with me;
Fight against those who fight against me. Take hold of shield
and buckler, and stand up for my help. Also draw out the spear,
and stop those who pursue me. Say to my soul, "I am your
salvation." Let those be put to shame and brought to dishonor
who seek after my life; Let those be turned back and brought to
confusion who plot my hurt. Let them be like chaff before the
wind, and let the angel of the Lord chase them. Let their way be
dark and slippery, and let the angel of the Lord pursue them...
And my soul shall be joyful in the Lord; It shall rejoice in His
salvation. All my bones shall say, "Lord, who is like You,
Delivering the poor from him who is too strong for him,
Yes, the poor and the needy from him who plunders him?"
(Psalm 35:1-5, 9, NKJV)

And He has given you tools to fight with:

A final word: Be strong in the Lord and in his mighty power.
Put on all of God's armor so that you will be able to stand firm
against all strategies of the devil. For we are not fighting against
flesh-and-blood enemies, but against evil rulers and authorities
of the unseen world, against mighty powers in this dark world,
and against evil spirits in the heavenly places. Therefore, put
on every piece of God's armor so you will be able to resist the
enemy in the time of evil. Then after the battle you will still be
standing firm. Stand your ground, putting on the belt of truth
and the body armor of God's righteousness. For shoes, put on the
peace that comes from the Good News so that you will be fully
prepared. In addition to all of these, hold up the shield of faith to
stop the fiery arrows of the devil. Put on salvation as your hel-

met, and take the sword of the Spirit, which is the word of God. Pray in the Spirit at all times and on every occasion. Stay alert and be persistent in your prayers for all believers everywhere (Ephesians 6: 10-18, NLT).

So take up your armor and fight, knowing:

The LORD himself goes before you and will be with you; he will never leave you nor forsake you. Do not be afraid; do not be discouraged (Deuteronomy 31:8, NIV).

And that He never expected you to fight in your own strength:

So he answered and said to me: "This is the word of the Lord to Zerubbabel: 'Not by might nor by power, but by My Spirit,' Says the Lord of hosts (Zechariah 4:6, NKJV).

CHAPTER 16: A NEW NAME

These Scars- July 2015
He makes beautiful what has been broken. Marks to
remind me. Words I did not leave unspoken.
Written in color. Things I thought I believed in. Each mark tells
a story. Each word was a chapter. I am not the same woman
that at that time sought after...
Something to make me stand out.
To make my confused stance clear at first impression. Now I
must be clear through my actions because He has made new my
every transgression.
Your Love is written on my heart. This ink bleeds through me
reminds me I need thee.
Lord may Your Love shine brighter through me illuminate even
the markings I feel have ruined me. May You use them to paint
a picture of a life You're still restoring. Of a soul that was desperately searching. Of a heart that was dead set on revolting...
This temple is tainted. This temple is painted. This temple is
Yours. It is the one You created.
And what You created is beautiful. Despite my attempts at home
improvement. Remind me it's the condition of the interior that
concerns You
And not the rebellious rendition of an imperfect creation...

One thing I have struggled with is the fact that I am covered with tattoos representing things I no longer stand for. My mentors had me read Acts when I first came back to Christ. Paul's encounter with Christ and transformation resonated so deeply with mine. It is an interesting place to be in when you are advocating for and representing something, in full belief that what you stand for is the right way. Only to have Jesus knock

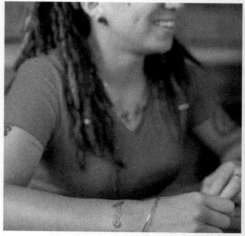

you off your horse, blind you, and tell you that *actually* you've been wrong for quite some time, and you're now going to stand for all things Jesus. So maybe I didn't get knocked off my horse and though my vision is terrible, I'm pretty sure I can still see, but that's what it felt like. And I couldn't be more thankful or feel more loved that He did. But it is scary. When I first came back to Him, I tried to find ways to cover these tattoos because I was, I suppose, ashamed of them.

Fear not; you will no longer live in shame. Don't be afraid; there is no more disgrace for you. You will no longer remember the shame of your youth and the sorrows of widowhood. For your Creator will be your husband; the LORD of Heaven's Armies is his name! He is your Redeemer, the Holy One of Israel, the God of all the earth. For the LORD has called you back from your grief— as though you were a young wife abandoned by her husband," says your God. "For a brief moment I abandoned you, but with great compassion I will take you back. In a

*burst of anger I turned my face away for a little while. But with
everlasting love I will have compassion on you," says the LORD,
your Redeemer. "Just as I swore in the time of Noah that I would
never again let a flood cover the earth, so now I swear that I will
never again be angry and punish you. For the mountains may
move and the hills disappear, but even then my faithful love for
you will remain. My covenant of blessing will never be broken,"
says the LORD, who has mercy on you (Isaiah 54:4-10, NLT).*

When people ask me if I am Muslim because of the star
and crescent or compliment my rainbow 'Coexist' tattoo,
I never know quite how to respond. I got it hoping people
would see it and wonder what I believed, because I hadn't a
clue at one point. I also hoped they would see the rainbow and
know that I was proudly gay. Now, when people ask, my answer usually begins with a smile as I recount where I was and
how far He has brought me. I am learning that these marks
tell a story and already have opened many doors to share with
others the transformative power of Jesus Christ, to share what
He has done in my life.

*...For the testimony of Jesus is the spirit of prophecy (Revela-
tion 19:10, NKJV).*

My prayer is that He continues to use them for His glory.
I may bear the markings of my past, but I am covered by a
larger marking, the blood of Jesus Christ.

*And they overcame him by the blood of the Lamb and by the
word of their testimony, and they did not love their lives to the
death (Revelation 12:11, NKJV).*

Deeper than the markings on my skin, were the markings on my heart. After years of being hurt and hurting others over and over and over again, one builds significant scar tissue. This becomes the barrier that allows you to deal with the pain, or rather pretend the gaping wound does not exist. The internal wounds were the shame and hurt I carried, not so much from being hurt as from realizing the damage I had caused in others' lives. Some who, initially had come to Christ through my witness, but watched me completely turn my back and then followed me as I encouraged them to do the same.

Some who I made promises to and did not keep. Some who I lied to in order to get what I wanted out of them, only to then pretend I never knew them after I did. Some I tried to convince that Jesus was a hoax and the Bible, a joke, not at all because I believed that. But because I desperately wanted to believe because I did not see how I could ever climb from the deep hole I continued to dig for myself. Remembering these events, these people, writing about this…brings back the pain. I have apologized to many people, and I don't expect a response or even that they still remember or care. I just want them to know I am sorry and that if I could re-do those interactions, I would do things very differently.

The enemy will try to use guilt and shame to constantly remind you of what you have done in your past, and to make you feel that you cannot change or move forward. In all honesty, you cannot. But when you have come to Christ and repented of your sins, that's it. You're forgiven. Satan has no hold on you, unless you dwell there or return. In God's book, you are made new.

"Come now, let's settle this," says the LORD. "Though your sins are like scarlet, I will make them as white as snow. Though

they are red like crimson, I will make them as white as wool (Isaiah 1:18, NLT).

So when the enemy comes to try and steal your joy and make you think you are worthless, remind him of this. You've settled the matter with the only One Who's opinion matters and therefore *there is no condemnation for those who belong to Christ Jesus (Romans 8:1, NLT).*

And the result of God's gracious gift is very different from the result of that one man's sin. For Adam's sin led to condemnation, but God's free gift leads to our being made right with God, even though we are guilty of many sins (Romans 5:16, NLT).

A New Name- August 2015
I don't want to go back there in fact I promised that I won't
All that's there is empty and broken how on earth am I seeing gold?
I didn't take five steps forward to take ten back even one or two and I'm completely off track suddenly listening to voices I know tell me lies suddenly what I know will only hurt me familiarity undisguised seems easier than getting back up easier than giving it another try
Thing is I've done what I tend to do when I get busy when I attempt to do this on my own when I don't make time to be in Your presence when I don't make Your heart my home
It was stupid of me to make that promise good thing You knew that the moment I did good thing You know me better than I do good thing You're loving and quick to forgive good thing You're not holding me to perfection good thing You're not holding me to my mistakes good thing You're here holding me when I can't hold it together good thing You're my savior my lifeboat my

strength.

Lord keep me close when I drift off I'm sorry, I didn't think I'd sailed out to sea I didn't realize how weak I had gotten didn't recognize I'd fallen asleep

It didn't faze me when I talked about my past as if it was my current my yesterday my today I didn't notice my senses were failing I let my busy let my guard down my carnal embraced I may not have acted out or rebelled in a way that was gaudy from the outside I'm sure I still seemed the same but inside my heart was slowly fading my soul starving my spirit thirsting for rain

I learned I can't promise not to fail because I'm falling but this time I'm asking You to please take my hand take my heart take my mind guard my senses remind me who I am in You remind me you have given me a new name.

This new name is tainted and trying this new name is weak and not so bold this new name is leaning on Your promise this new name has a story to be told

This new name is asking forgiveness though I may fall give me the courage to take hold of this new name and all of Your loving kindness, You're my Faithful Forever...my Redeemer, my Hope.

CHAPTER 17: LIFE NOW

Journal- 2015
> I hurt a lot of people.
> I led a lot of people astray.

My own heart and soul had been ripped apart, mostly by my own doing.

Eventually I got to this place.

This place of complete brokenness, so deep that I realized if I were to break anymore I might not be able to recover.

He met me here.

Well, He had always been pursuing me....but it was in this place I made the life altering decision to take His hand.

I thought I had to get my life together, take care of the mess I had made during my rebellion.

The thought of having to fix my mess was so overwhelming and very impossible.

The reason this coming back to Him has been different from all of the other times I tried, is because this time I learned not to try. I learned that He offers His hand and asks you to come to Him as you are.

Don't go back and try to pick up the pieces because you will fail. Allow Him to carry you and His love will fix the deepest most intimate places in your life that you thought couldn't be *reached.*

Come as you are and allow Me to not just put the pieces back together, but to completely undo you so that I can put you back together again, a whole, new creation in Me.

A few months after coming back to Christ, I had a dream that really had me bothered when I woke up the next morning. It was the strangest thing, because usually I remember them very clearly, or I just know I had a dream but can remember nothing at all. When I woke up, all I could remember was the beginning of the dream, it seemed as if the rest had just been cut off.

I was on what seemed to be a retreat and I was standing outside of the building we were staying in. There was a homeless woman crying on the steps leading up to the building. As I watched her, my heart broke, so I approached her to try to see how I could help. She asked for a hug, and as I went to hug her she transformed right before my eyes into this beautiful, beautiful woman. She all of the sudden smelled like perfume and had nice clothes on. She began whispering to me, and pulling me closer, trying to kiss me. I remember my thoughts and feelings being at war with each other, but it stopped there. I could not remember if I ran or stayed.

This particular day was a rough day at work, and this dream, or what I could remember from it, had me feeling discouraged and defeated. I thought I had come so far- why would I be dreaming something like this? Suddenly, out of nowhere, I remembered a little bit more. I could see myself running. I ran. I didn't stay. I still could not tell if this was the end, but I was relieved that I ran. That night, as I was getting ready for bed, I remembered the end of the dream. I was standing in front of a mirror, but my face didn't look like mine- it was swollen, seemingly beat up. And as I stood there looking at myself, I was speaking truth over the situation. "Satan you have no say, no control, I rebuke you in the Name of Jesus. My identity is in Him, alone. His promises are yes and Amen. I am not bound by this sin. I am victorious in Him. You will not win. I may be bruised, but I am not defeated."

I have been asked why this change is different than any of the other times I tried to return to Christ. What if this is just a phase? I would answer that I know this is a lasting change, because my perspective has changed. My heart has changed. There are many things and people in this world who are capable of influencing and manipulating someone's choices and/or behavior, but there is nothing and no one that can completely alter perspective, completely change someone's

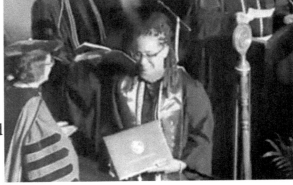

heart. If it weren't for God pursuing my heart, it would make no sense to have gone through all of the heartache of leaving what had become my way of life and identity.

He sought me out, and gave me His peace and love like I had never experienced. When I acknowledged Him in my life and began asking for more of Him, He began convicting me of not only homosexuality, but of so many other sins I had opened my life up to. He not only convicted me, but he gave me the strength to completely walk away. I repented and walked away from all kinds of sexual sin, from drunkenness, bad language, stealing, lying, and cheating. Things I never even gave a second thought about doing, all of a sudden became so clearly not okay.

I began to notice aspects of my character long forgotten, 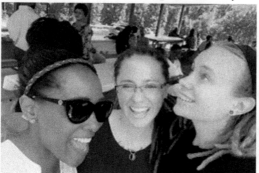 coming back to life. Suddenly it was easier to have patience. Suddenly it was easier to love and see hope in situations that before had seemed hopeless. Suddenly, I found myself reaching out to friends and family because I was not so completely consumed with my own life. Suddenly, I was singing to the top of my lungs in my car on my way to work like a crazy person because that is just how much joy and love consumed my heart.

Like I said, this change initially meant I had to stop doing a lot of things. I intentionally stopped listening to a lot of music, watching certain shows and movies, going to certain places altogether. Those are the things I had to not do in order to guard my heart so that He could heal it. Eventually I got to this place where I no longer felt like I was giving anything up. It no longer felt like sacrifice, and it never was. Jesus giving His life for mine- that was sacrifice. This was surrender. Surrender of my sin and my idols, of my heart and my mind.

I have had moments where I do let fear get the best of me. So that question, "how do you know this is lasting?" used to worry me, because I questioned my strength, and the extent of change in my life. I knew I had walked away from a lot, and I prayed for God to help break ties, and naturally after about ten declined offers, people just stopped inviting me to do things I used to do and to go places I used to go. In the beginning, it was hard to say no, and I prayed that people would just not ask so I wouldn't even have to. Over the past few months, starting with that dream, I feel like God has been showing me just how far He has brought me. It is no longer hard to say no, in fact, those things are no longer appealing. I can think about places and people and pray for them rather than dwell on what was lost. There is truly nothing we could ever give up that could compare to what He gave up for us and what we gain in Him- His unconditional, redeeming love, eternally.

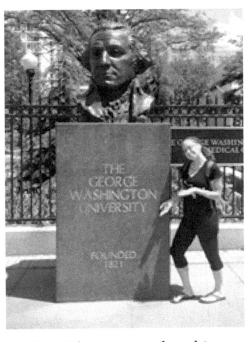

What does being "free" or walking in freedom look like? I have told you what I no longer do, but what do I do? Before coming back to Christ, I was under the impression that life as a Christian, with a list of "do's and don'ts", was a boring way to live. This was another thing that Satan used to try to bring me down in the beginning. I knew what not to do, but if you asked me how I was going to fill that time- all I knew was I was going to pray and read my Bible. Now, I don't know anybody whose day solely consists of praying and reading the Word. I'm sure there are people; I just don't know them. And right now, that actually sounds like a pretty amazing day.

However, when I first came back to Christ, the thought of that sounded extremely boring. My mentors taught me the importance of filling my time with fellowship- firstly with God and also with other believers. As mentioned earlier, this part is so key. There was one point where I was going to a different fellowship/small group every night of the week. As I am working full-time and in grad school, I soon found this to be quite impossible, but I was so scared of having any free time to myself to mess up. There must be a balance. And He will lead you to the right fellowship. Fellowship with Him comes first. I have also begun running again. This used to be something I loved, but after taking up smoking and drinking, it no longer felt so great. It feels good to run again.

My young adult group has multiple fellowship opportunities and there is always something going on at church. I get together with my friends from church for dinner or coffee and fellowship often. I have discovered plenty of Christian music that I love. I was a Hip-Hop fan and I loved to dance. I found out about Christian Hip-Hop- there are some incredible artists out there, and I still dance- I just dance for Jesus now! I can't get enough worship. I play my guitar. I write music,

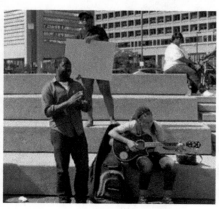

poetry, journal entries. I am involved with evangelism at church and we have a big evangelism event once a month.

Recently, we went to downtown Baltimore and I had the opportunity to play my guitar and worship while we passed out pizza and prayed with people. I spend more time with my grandparents and on Skype with my family in Africa. Then, there is grad school, which takes up a good bit of my time too. Honestly, I find myself constantly running out of hours in the day. And I am truly at peace and joyful in all of these things, so long as He is at the center.

Therefore, since we have been made right in God's sight by faith, we have peace with God because of what Jesus Christ our Lord has done for us. Because of our faith, Christ has brought us into this place of undeserved privilege where we now stand, and we confidently and joyfully look forward to sharing God's glory. We can rejoice, too, when we run into problems and trials, for we know that they help us develop endurance. And endurance develops strength of character, and character strengthens our confident hope of salvation. And this hope will not lead to disappointment. For we know how dearly God loves us, because he has given us the Holy Spirit to fill our hearts with his love (Romans 5:1-5, NLT).

The Holy Spirit has filled my heart with love. My heart is overwhelmed daily by His presence and by the love shown through my brothers and sisters in Christ. Love was something that had become very warped in my mind, especially romantical love, which is hard, because that kind of love is meant to mirror the love Christ has for us. I believe that the gift of having a husband or a wife are meant for God to more tangibly demonstrate His love for us. I am not sure what the future holds, but I know that if it is His plan for me to be married, He will and maybe already is preparing my heart. I am not concerned about this. I know that He is good. I know that He will also work in the heart of whoever that hypothetical person may be, to love me for and despite everything.

I no longer see my past as baggage. I see it as a redemption story. He took the load and in exchange gave me new life, peace, and unending joy through His love. Yes, I was once an on-fire kid for Jesus, but I was cocky, immature, and I never truly understood who I was in Him. It was all about me, because I needed to be affirmed. Perhaps, I had to go through all of this in order to realize how much I need Him. Also, if I hadn't gone through the fire, I would not know how dangerous it is to even get close. After having been in the fire, I know I do not want to go back there. I see now how many times He held me when many situations may have caused a great deal more harm than they did. I would not be able to stand as I do now, and my love for Him would not be what it is today.

Just as He had to make Joseph a slave, a servant, a prisoner, before He could use Him as a leader, I believe sometimes, He doesn't cause things to happen per-say, but He allows us to choose certain paths and to experience them fully so that we might understand, fully, why He wants otherwise for us. Why He wants His children to live Holy just as He is Holy. Why He longs that we would just choose Him and trust that He only wants what is best for us. However, no matter what path we choose, He is there in the midst of our mess gently calling us back to Him, and developing our character along the way.

And I am certain that God, who began the good work within you, will continue his work until it is finally finished on the day when Christ Jesus returns (Philippians 1:6, NLT).

I realize in writing and sharing this story, there will be people who do not agree or like what I have to say. But I cannot help but share- I cannot hold it in. He has completely changed my life, and I will never be the same because of Him. I cannot go back to my old life, nor do I want to. There is something about experiencing Him that does not allow you to. Once you realize what you gain in Him, once you catch a glimpse of His perfect love for you, which allows you to begin to see yourself the way He does, everything else becomes trivial.

So though my flesh is weak, I know that He is my strength, and I know that His plans for my life are good. I know that there may be persecution. I realize there may be a time where my convictions, my love, and my stand for Jesus Christ may cost more than simply giving up and walking away from things that were not good for me in the first place. But He gave it all for me, so I pray for the courage and the love to give nothing less than my all to and for Him.

For I am not ashamed of this Good News about Christ. It is the power of God at work, saving everyone who believes—the Jew first and also the Gentile. This Good News tells us how God makes us right in his sight. This is accomplished from start to finish by faith. As the Scriptures say, "It is through faith that a righteous person has life." (Romans 1:16-17, NLT)

I am so thankful He didn't give up on me. I would have given up on me. Good thing I'm not God, right? It's so easy to think that He thinks like us, because we cannot imagine anything else. If you are someone struggling with homosexuality, please know there is a way out. Please take courage in the fact that He used the very relationship I was in to bring me and my ex back to Him. He has a plan. His plan will prevail. He has already won and He is fighting for and with you. He will fortify you through other believers, so don't isolate yourself.

A few months after coming back to Christ, I had the honor of meeting a lady, who is now a spiritual mom to me. When I first started to fall away 8 years ago, God made it clear to her, though she lived on the other side of the world and in a state I had never even been close to, that she was to stand in the gap for me. That she was to pray on my behalf, no matter how long it took. When she told me her story and I realize how God used her, my family members, and so many others to pray and fight the spiritual battles I was unaware were raging around me, it leaves me in complete and absolute awe. He takes every detail into account. And He has prayer warriors, Nehemiah's, standing in the gap for you, too.

Do not be afraid to be vulnerable. His heart breaks when yours breaks, you are His treasure, His lamb, His most prized possession. And don't beat yourself up when at first your feelings don't align with what you know to be true. Coming out of a lifestyle that has been your identity is painful and involves a healing process that does not happen overnight. Remember that His Word trumps feelings, always. And the more you seek His face and learn to trust His heart, the more you will start to find joy in living in Him, as your desires begin to align with His.

He will never stop pursuing your heart. He loves you with a love unending, unconditional. He will never leave nor forsake you. Cling to Him- I know it hurts. It is going to hurt. Tell Him how you feel, how you hurt, cry out to Him. He will not leave you to deal with it on your own. Jesus is drawn to brokenness, He is Healer. He will meet you in this place and He will strengthen your heart till you can stand. Seek fellowship, as accountability and support is crucial in our Christian walk, regardless of our individual battles. Do not be afraid to reach out, to take His hand, to fall into His arms. I promise it will be the best decision you ever make.

I have told you all this so that you may have peace in me. Here on earth you will have many trials and sorrows. But take heart, because I have overcome the world (John 16:33, NLT)

If you are a parent or a friend, know that prayer is powerful. Do not stop praying. Speak truth, in love. I did not take it very well when I was in the middle of it all, but looking back I am so grateful I had people in my life who loved me enough to speak truth. My heart was hardened then, but seeds were planted. When I finally decided to stop fighting against Him and my heart began to soften, these seeds, which had taken root throughout the years, began to spring to life as if they had just been planted. Pray for God to direct how and when and what you say. He can and will

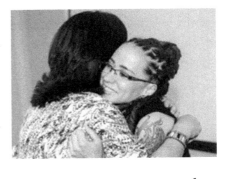

use you to bring your loved ones back to Him. Set boundaries, but love your children where they are at and pray without ceasing.

If your prayer life is something that has been lacking in the past, let this be the thing that turns you into a prayer warrior. I cannot stress enough the power of prayer. Gather together with other parents and set up prayer sessions where you meet to specifically war for your children. My mom started meeting weekly with two of my friends' moms when I first began to struggle and they have each seen their children come out of lifestyles and struggles that many do not ever make it out of. God is surely faithful.

And He responds when we cry out to Him. I often wish I could see what exactly goes on in the spiritual realm when a prayer is released by a heart desperate for a move of God.

So He said to them, "This kind can come out by nothing but prayer and fasting (Mark 9:29, NKJV).

But these things I plan won't happen right away. Slowly, surely, steadily, the time approaches when the vision will be fulfilled. If it seems slow, do not despair, for these things will surely come to pass. Just be patient! They will not be overdue a single day! (Habakkuk 2:3, TLB)

If you are a pastor or a leader in a church, facing pressure to go against what you know in your heart of hearts is truth, even from members of the church, I want to encourage you in your stance on maintaining a Biblical standard when it comes to same sex relationships and marriages. I am not alone in following Christ out of a lifestyle that many in the world think is crazy talk to "come out of". I didn't think it was possible. I truly believed this was who I was- it was my entire identity. It's a good thing we serve a God Who created us and therefore knows us inside and out. He knows us better than anyone, even ourselves.

It is not His plan for us to live in sin- sin that is so clearly and lovingly dealt with in the Bible. As His body, He desires and commands that we uphold His word. That we be the light, through love, to the many that are still lost and so in need of the same saving grace we have received. How can we offer this hope, this salvation, this freedom, if we, when facing pressure, criticism, even persecution, do not abide by His Word? We are warned that the world will not like us (1 John 3:13). We are warned that we will be persecuted. But we are also told that in standing for Him, we are blessed and have reason to rejoice (Matt 5:10, Luke 6:22).

Beloved, do not be surprised at the fiery trial when it comes upon you to test you, as though something strange were happening to you. But rejoice insofar as you share Christ's sufferings, that you may also rejoice and be glad when his glory is revealed. If you are insulted for the name of Christ, you are blessed, because the Spirit of glory and of God rests upon you (1 Peter 4:12-14, ESV)

The time for the church to stand for His truth, in its entirety, is now. If His church won't stand, who will?

Journal- October 2015
I wish everyone I know and love could see and truly understand how meaningless everything is if Jesus is not the center. The past 7 years of my life did not reflect that- no- quite the contrary...but the past year...He has become so very real to me. More real than anything or anyone I have ever known. And this urgency...this calling...His pursuit of your heart is the most beautiful thing you will ever experience, apart from actually running...or falling, as was my case...into the arms of Love, Himself. Jesus is the One and only way. No, I'm not closed minded...in fact my mind heart and soul have never been more open to truth. I did not leave my old way of life behind because I was not "happy" or because it was no longer comfortable. I walked away...and it hurt. More than any hurt I have ever felt. But the calling, the urgency, His love is so great...I couldn't continue living that way. When I finally stopped to evaluate, to feel...to let the numbness I built up over the years melt away and felt that

deep and dark emptiness of a life I was trying to live in my own strength, using all of that strength to needlessly push away the One who only ever wanted to fight for me never against me...I realized that more than anything and no matter what may come...I was and am and always will be in need of a Savior. In need of redemption. In need of Jesus. And once you truly know the good news, because friends- it is the BEST news you will ever hear...once you know and have experienced even a glimpse of what this means...of the absolute unending and unconditional love He has for you...You will never want to go back either. I can promise you that. When you know the truth...when you have the answer...the only thing to do is to share it. It would be so selfish not to. So all of that to simply say this: He loves you.

He loves you.

He loves you.

And He wants you to know there is more to life.

Let Him be your everything.

I promise you He is worth it.

This Love is everything.

EPILOGUE

Blog: Full Circle 4.4.16

My heart is so very overwhelmed. The doors He is opening. The doors He has closed and the ones He is continuing to close…the old creaky ones that try to sneak their way open…He gently seals shut but not without my permission. He is a perfect Gentleman. The Perfect Gentleman. And I am thankful He is closing off those areas…but not before He has had me walk through them…sometimes crawling, sometimes scared stiff- frozen in place, gently encouraging me to keep going as I slowly and longingly attempt taking steps backwards…steps back to what was for so long so very comfortable. He has and is still healing the broken places, illuminating every corner and crevice and at times He has had to carry me through the rooms that hold the memories that I could not bear to sort through. And He didn't ask me to. He simply called me to surrender my heart. And never once chastised me for being fearful and resorting back to my once familiar comfort zone…which, to my constant amazement, no longer feels so familiar or comfortable.

Remembering who I was and where I've been. Who I've hurt and words I've spoken…that is uncomfortable. But I am learning that there is surely a great difference between Godly sorrow and shameful sorrow…I do not regret my past. I am wholeheartedly and sincerely repentant for the pain I caused. I now know that if I had not lived in the fire for 8 years, I would have no idea what it means to have unshakeable faith. I would have no real understanding of why it is absolutely necessary to live a holy life. To be set apart. To purposefully and intentionally stay as far away from the fire as possible, because the heat is dangerous. I once thought I could live completely for Christ, and still have one foot kind of, sort of, sometimes, partially in the world. I didn't see a problem with this. But then again, at that time I also had absolutely no clue I was even losing my balance, slowly slipping, until after I had fallen flat on my face, unable to see through the fog to pinpoint where exactly it was I had even fallen from.

I had the privilege of witnessing one of God's most beautiful creations last week…and as I stood and stared at the Grand Canyon before me….at the deep valley below…as I willed the butterflies in my tummy to settle…I thought to myself… it once felt like I had fallen to the bottom of the Grand Canyon…and I'm pretty sure it felt like what it must feel like to look up…thousands of feet above you at a cliff you had at one point so carelessly frolicked around on. It hurts to see others frolic on this cliff. It hurts to see the ones you love willingly, despite your direction, your scorn…walk towards the fire. It hurts to watch those you love hurt themselves. It hurts to see someone, who reminds you so very much of yourself, making the same mistakes. I often wonder what I would have listened to as a teenager…who I would have listened to. And quite frankly, I still have no answer to that. When your heart has been hardened…mostly by your own doing…even the sharpest arrows cannot seem to break through.

I have learned that God doesn't always operate in sharp

and forceful. Like I said…perfect Gentleman. It is and will be the seeds, lovingly and gently tossed, in prayer that they might find whatever fertile ground remains…that break ground and dig their roots deep into a heart that seems to receive nothing and no one. They will blossom in time and serve as constant, often annoying, reminders that there is nothing in this world that will ever separate or put an end to the perfect love of a Father Who, though He has an entire flock, does not stop pursuing His one sheep who has wondered away. A Father Who sent His Son to die so that one sheep could return and know Love, Himself. A Father who loves this one more than any of their friends or family members ever could. All they are called to do is to endlessly lift up their lost one in prayer…often times, prayer that is weak and shaky…barely audible…and painfully broken.

The Lord is close to the brokenhearted; He rescues those whose spirits are crushed (Psalm 34:18, NLT).

I was once this sheep. And I truly believe that it was because of these prayers, uttered by warriors who stood in the gap and fought for me on their knees, that the battles that were waged and ensuing constantly around me though I had not a clue, did not end in the enemy's favor. It is truly surreal to be in a place now where I can stand in the gap for someone else. Because when one of us is lost and hurting, we all hurt. And when it seems there is no hope and nothing is getting through, please remember that there was a time I accepted that I was a lost cause. But when I was too numb to hear His voice and too blind to see truth, others spoke on His behalf, saw truth for me, and did not give up the fight. And though I got tired of fighting, there was never a second He gave up fighting for me. His love knows no bounds. Not even the hardest heart can keep Him out. And He is already victorious. Even if it means we have to go through the fire sometimes to see it.

My sheep listen to my voice; I know them, and they follow me. I give them eternal life, and they will never perish. No one can snatch them away from me, for my Father has given them to me, and he is more powerful than anyone else. No one can snatch them from the Father's hand. The Father and I are one (John 10:27-30, NLT).

Song- Ransomed Heart
This ransomed heart here beating
A soul made new, no longer pleading
For grace I never earned
For love I don't deserve
Your mercies are new every day
The point where grace and fear meet
I throw myself at your feet
So much to say
Thoughts that replay
But I can't speak
Lead me, guide me
Be in front and beside me
Lead me, guide me
Let Your gentle Love remind me...
You said come all you weary
I'll give you rest if you seek Me
Lay down your pride
And all you hide behind
I have won, you are Mine

I will shout for joy and sing Your praises,
for You have ransomed me!
Psalms 71:23

About Gabrielle

Gabrielle Rehmeyer is a community health nurse in Baltimore, currently working towards her master's in public health to further pursue her love for working with vulnerable populations. She is involved in her church, CAC Bethel Baltimore, as well as Bethel Campus Fellowship, a ministry dedicated to the discipleship of high schoolers, college students, and young adults. Her heart's desire is to share the redemptive power of Christ, to help broken hearts find their home, their healing, their freedom, and their identity in His love and saving grace.

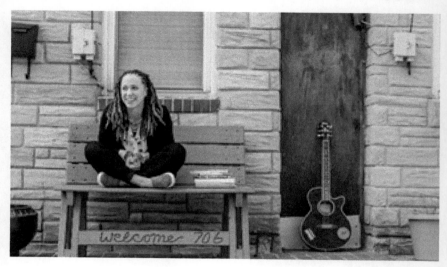

First Love Media
Tulsa, OK

"Serving the Christian church with materials for spiritual growth, deeper worship, and victorious living."

www.FirstLoveMedia.com

... for the earth shall be full of the knowledge of the LORD, as the waters cover the sea (Isaiah 11:9).

CPSIA information can be obtained
at www.ICGtesting.com
Printed in the USA
BVHW01s2250150118
505308BV00007BA/23/P